Praise for Dorothy

"Dorothy is a life coach. She is abou... ...together an action plan for setting up the interval steps to get you where you're going, setting realistic goals—and she is good at it."

—**Dr. Phil McGraw**, the *Dr. Phil* **show**

"A few hours of Dorothy Breininger's time saves me hundreds of hours of my own time, while bringing me greatly increased efficiency and peace of mind."

—**Dr. Jared Diamond**, **Pulitzer Prize winner**
bestselling author, *Guns, Germs and Steel*

"My early success was built on creating sexy, carefree, unstructured hairstyles for men and women. My staying power is due to structure and organization in my life. Dorothy's book will give you what you need to achieve that carefree feeling with the long-term staying power for success."

—**José Eber, world's most acclaimed hairstylist**

"Dorothy Breininger is winning a squeaky-clean reputation as a clutter-buster without equal. A five-foot-tall former gymnast and former executive assistant to deans at Northeastern University in Boston and the University of California, Ms. Breininger has morphed herself into a compact white tornado."

—*Christian Science Monitor*

"In her book, Breininger says what is eating you today can serve up heaps of self-destructive habits that can last a lifetime. And the world's best makeover will not alleviate the pain unless you face your stuff."

—*Warner Center News*

"Some people go to Bali on vacation. I just call Dorothy!"

—**Susan Beckman, artist**

"Dorothy Breininger can turn your 'To Do' list into an 'It's Done' list!"

—*Organize* **magazine**

"Dorothy Breininger knows a thing or two about motivation and goal setting."

—*Rapid City Journal*

"For years Dorothy and her staff have organized my business and my life. For me, Dorothy is like a monthly vitamin, which ensures my personal and business success."

—Roxanne Davis, attorney

"Dorothy Breininger and her team were amazing to work with—they took mountains of paper and created organized files. We no longer feel overwhelmed by the sheer volume of information we process."

—Southern California Edison

"Nobody appreciates a high-class pigsty like Dorothy Breininger. Her tales from the upper crust of disorganization will send you jogging to the nearest Staples."

—*Forbes* magazine

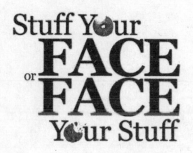

Stuff Your FACE or FACE Your Stuff

Lose Weight By
Decluttering Your Life

Dorothy
"The Organizer"
Breininger, as seen on the *Hoarders*®
series on A&E®

Health Communications, Inc.
Deerfield Beach, Florida

www.hcibooks.com

Library of Congress Cataloging-in-Publication Data

Breininger, Dorothy K.
  Stuff your face or face your stuff : the organized approach to lose weight by decluttering your life / Dorothy K. Breininger.
     pages cm
  ISBN-13: 978-0-7573-1737-8 (Paperback)
  ISBN-10: 0-7573-1737-5 (Paperback)
  ISBN-13: 978-0-7573-1738-5 (ePub)
  ISBN-10: 0-7573-1738-3 (ePub)
  1. Weight loss—Psychological aspects.   2. Orderliness—Health aspects.
3. Compulsive hoarding.   I. Title.
  RJ506.E18B74 2013
  616.85'26—dc23

                                                                    2013011149

©2013 Dorothy Breininger

Publisher: Health Communications, Inc.
            3201 S.W. 15th Street
            Deerfield Beach, FL 33442–8190

Cover photo of Dorothy Breininger by Keith Muyan
Cover design by Dane Wesolko
Interior design and formatting by Lawna Patterson Oldfield

CONTENTS

*There are people who come along in life
to ensure you are cared for. My business partners,
Debby and Ken Bitticks, care for me and others deeply.
They have made it their life's work to listen, advise,
and then mobilize themselves and others to create solutions
for our greater success, happiness, and good health.
I dedicate this book to them because of their unrelenting support
of me over the years. In every case with me and with others,
they always seek to do the right thing. Bottom line:
they show understanding and kindness to all
those who come into contact with them.*

ACKNOWLEDGMENTS

For once, I'm going to do it right and put my mom first on the list. Thank you for becoming such a graceful parent. As we age together, I have finally found a way for my temperamental self to love you and accept your love in return. You are remarkable.

I would like to thank my business partners, Debby and Ken Bitticks, Lynn and Steven Benson, and all of our Delphi staff, investors, bankers, attorneys, vendors, and clients who supported our company—especially during the darkest days of the recession. I would like to thank my sister Pat, who was my guide for this book: her intelligence and confidence helped me to turn the corner in creating this book's success. I would like to thank my sister Chris and my brother, Edd, for their willingness to overlook my egotistic nature and love me anyway. I would like to thank my contributing writers: Val Sgro, Debby Bitticks, Lynn Benson, Pat Brady, MaryAnne Bennie, Karen Koedding, Dr. Charlene Underhill Miller, Kipling Solid, Timolin Langin, Dee Dee Wilson Barton, and, most especially, our very own Gillian Drake. I would also like to thank my stand-behind-me, stand-beside-me, pull-me-up-from-under friends Martina Koerner (my cousin), Nancy Korn, Jeanette Brennan, Dr. Kevin Brennan, Diana Thatcher, Amy Siu, John Hanley, Andrea Eitland, Ed Thein, and Valerie Pugliese.

I am grateful to my mentors: David Boyd, Abdelmomen Afifi, Marty Feldman, Tony Robbins, Jack Canfield, Mark Victor Hansen, Denise Kovac, Kristin Maclaughlin, Sharma Bennett, Winston Alt, and the staff and course leaders of Landmark Education. Of course, I must thank my publisher, Peter Vegso; PR guru Kim Weiss; and my writing Sherpa, Allison Janse. Gratitude also goes to my wise copy editors, Cathy Slovensky and Bob Land. Hooray for my amazing book publicists Gretchen Koss and Meghan Walker. Thank you to A&E® Network and Foxtel in Australia, the Screaming Flea Production team of *Hoarders*®, and all the clients, experts, and production crew on the show *Hoarders*®. Finally, I thank the thousands of professional organizing experts who belong to the National Association of Professional Organizers (NAPO), the Institute for Challenging Disorganization, and the millions of anonymous members who belong to the 12-step world.

INTRODUCTION:
How to Use This Book

The ultimate goal of this book is to inspire you to take action in one or more parts of your life that you may be avoiding—especially if you are overeating or obsessing about food because of it. My guess is that you, like me, have tried countless numbers of books, diets, or programs and still find yourself wondering why you continue to gain weight and muddle up your life. Perhaps that is why you are reading this book. No matter what your age, you realize that you need to find an answer—not just to the weight gain but to other parts of your life that you just don't talk about. You see, I have learned that the messier my home gets, the more my bills pile up, the more phone calls I avoid, or the more times I'm late to appointments, it is seemingly linked to my overeating. It's the "stuff" we don't want to talk about that is causing us to overeat or make unhealthy choices. Because I am a professional organizer, I liken it to lifting up the clutter to see what's underneath—whether it's others' or my own. This book helps you do that.

According to new data from the NPD Group, a market research firm, the number of people interested in dieting is down and the number of people interested in losing weight is up. What to do? Create your own plan. Harry Balzer, NPD's chief industry analyst, says that the most popular diet is one that people say "they made up, one they call 'my own diet.'" Balzer further reports that about a third of people follow a plan of their own.[1]

Well, that's just what happened to me. Trial and error. Determination followed by complacency. Embarrassment then enlightenment. In my five decades on this planet, I have been able to transform my major mistakes into incredible insights for myself. I no longer want to do it all alone. I want to share it with you. Whether you're in a relationship that's not working, you're avoiding paying bills, you're stepping over too much clutter on the floor, or you're stuffing your face with food, today you can begin to take a look at how you, like me, can face your stuff.

1

STUFFING IT:
A Recipe for Disaster

I t was during my third season filming *Hoarders*®. I was asked to fly to a bustling Midwestern town to work with a woman who hoards toys (for kids who've long grown up), clothes (that no longer fit), and more than a dozen goats, several dogs, a bunch of chickens and roosters, a few cats, and a couple of birds. The woman, Maybelline, lives on a lovely manicured street and owns a large parcel of land, which, because of an old zoning law, allows for farm animals. Nearby suburban neighbors don't approve of Maybelline's hoard and don't like the look of her property. They complain of a dilapidated home with holes, overgrown brush, mishmash fencing, and farm animals roaming. Neighbors grumble at being interrupted by roosters announcing the day before the manufactured alarm clocks do. The neighbors roll their eyes when they have to swerve their cars around another loud and boisterous breakaway goat, and they resent the hoard of unstartable cars, immoveable boats, campers with broken windows, and wheel-less motorcycles that cover the front and back yards. Maybelline loves her goats even though they have chewed through the exterior siding and insulation of the house, through the interior walls, and into her back bedroom.

When I arrived on location with the show's therapist, Dr. Zasio, I met Maybelline and three of her goats in that bedroom; as I approached her, I gave Maybelline my usual hug and I could sense her warmth and willingness. I was reminded of the days when my dad, the town banker, was a guardian for some folks in my hometown of Richland Center, Wisconsin. He would take me with him on Saturday mornings and I had the chance to meet many of his clients—some of whom exhibited hoarding behavior. Holding my hand, my dad taught me as a seven-year-old to be very polite, keep any hurtful remarks to myself, and be interested in what they were saying. Today, every time I visit a client with hoarding problems, I feel my dad is with me. I asked Maybelline about her hoarding, focusing on some important questions: Are you a perfectionist? Does the "stuff" remind you of happier times? Have you experienced anxiety or depression in your lifetime?

This time, although I was talking with Maybelline, I began having an internal dialogue with my 200-pound self: *"Dorothy, are you a perfectionist?" "Heck, yeah! I was a gymnast for years, striving for a perfect 10—no mistakes!" "Dorothy, is there any anxiety or depression you don't want to talk about?" "I don't want to admit it, but yes. My sister was diagnosed with stage 4 cancer and I need to help her with her mortgage. My mentally challenged cousin has just come to live with us; I've moved in with my mom, sister, and cousin to help with the bills and the caregiving. I am working around the clock. I am depressed and anxious, and I am eating nonstop to cope."*

While my exterior self remained kind, loving, and professional, for the first time in my life, I was experiencing a shift in my own authentic, true self. As I was asking questions of Maybelline, I found myself answering them right along with her. In the midst of my internal verbal volley, I heard Maybelline again, talking about her need to cope—how she hoarded things because it brought her comfort. Was I hearing her story about hoarding or *my* story about overeating? As she explained that the toys and the clothes reminded her of happier times, I floated back to my own thoughts: *Yes, I'm attached to ice cream because it reminds me of my father. When he was alive we would go for ice cream in the evenings, and it was such a happy time for me. My cousin and I used to buy penny candy and play for hours at a time.* I yearned for those carefree days.

Stop! I don't believe this! I thought. I excused myself from Maybelline's presence and ran out in tears to the television production tent out front. I rarely cry on the set, but during my conversation with Maybelline, I realized that I was a hoarder, too. While I wasn't hoarding *things*, I was hoarding food—sugar, flour, and excess quantities of junk food on my body! In that moment, I saw that I was no different from Maybelline. She was buying, collecting, and hoarding stuff to fill a void, lessen anxiety, and reconnect with happier times in life—and so was I. I had developed this habit over the years to soothe myself, and it was identical to the behavior of my hoarding clients.

Maybelline and I sat down and designed new goals and dreams for her. She agreed to fix her camper and replace hoarding with traveling and adventure. We mended the goat-chewed holes in her house, and we substituted trash, soiled clothes, and old food and electronics lying about the house with artwork depicting mountains and eagles. We brought in soft blankets and rugs in outdoorsy colors and placed pine-scented candles throughout her home, reinforcing her dream of camping in the remote forests of North America. We also encouraged Maybelline to apologize to her neighbors, show them how we were dismantling the auto-parts division in her front yard, and let them know she intended to build proper fencing for the animals.

As I found with Maybelline and my own transformation, letting go of our "stuff" is often an emotional task as well as a physical one. But we can get there if we face it head-on.

Just as I excavate people from their homes and help them learn new habits, you can excavate the clutter around you and within you and learn new, healthier habits, too. *But first you need to understand that some of your issues about food may be more about emotional cravings than physical ones.*

The Disappearing Husband

Five, 5:30, 6:00 PM. He's not showing up. I've got family visiting from out of town and my husband has left us all waiting. We promised to meet at the house and head out to a Moroccan restaurant for dinner. He's usually on time. What's the matter with him? How could he let me down? How inconsiderate! He's embarrassing me! The least he could do is call!

Six-thirty, 7:00, 7:30 PM. Maybe something is wrong. I'll cancel the dinner reservations and we'll order in. But really, should I be worried? I dialed his cell phone for the seventeenth time in just a couple of hours' time.

Eight, 8:30, 9:00 PM. What do you say to family members who are looking at you funny when your husband doesn't come home when he's supposed to? My embarrassment had hit its height, but concern and worry started overtaking it. More calls to his cell phone. A call to his boss. Nothing.

Nine-thirty, 10:00, 10:30 PM. I turned to my sister Chris and niece, Morgen, and asked if they thought I should call the police or hospitals to see if something serious had happened to Bob. Despite our ups and downs, he always called—didn't he? Well, no. He didn't always call, but I ignored those times; they weren't as extreme as this. He had never done this to me when guests were involved. I called the hospitals and highway safety; no reports to their knowledge. I needed to inquire with the police directly.

Eleven, 11:30 PM, 12:00 midnight. I nervously got dressed and made my way to the police department to file a missing person's report. Not having done such a thing in my life, I didn't realize that it was too soon to do so. You mean seven hours of "no contact" didn't automatically make you a missing person? I was not able to file a report, so being my anxious self, I asked the officer on duty a slew of questions: Could he check the system for possible car accidents? Did he have a way to access hospital reports? Could he pull up my husband's car license plate number and track him? Tired of me and my questions, the officer had one question for me.

"Do you think your husband might be having a relationship with another woman?" he asked.

Well, put me in a boxing ring with gloves and a mouth guard and watch me fall to the floor in a total knockout! What? I'm shaking my head like a wet dog with water flying off my face as it goes from side to side! Huh?

"Well, no," I answered, embarrassed and ashamed. The officer could see he had made his point, and he offered a conciliatory "Why don't you just head home and try to get some sleep? I'm sure you'll hear from him. Hang in there."

I drove home in a fog, walked into the house where family members were still gathered in support of my missing-husband dilemma, and the phone rang. It was 1:30 AM. It was Bob. The first words were, "Dor, I only have a one-minute call. You need to find the best divorce attorney you can and divorce me, and could you call my brother and let him know I'm in jail for six felony counts? I need his help." I barely got another sentence in before asking the location of the jail where Bob was being held, then the phone went dead. I've only seen those scenarios in the movies, but now I understood that when you only get a minute to make a collect call, they aren't kidding. In that minute, the life I knew collapsed around me, and in the days afterward, my mind started searching for clues about my sixteen-year relationship with Bob. I knew I needed to face up to all the stuff I had ignored, pretended about, and lied about—to myself and others. I was in an unhealthy marriage and I needed to come clean. It would be years before I could admit my part not just in my marriage to Bob but about my entire life.

Some people hide behind booze. Some people gamble to over-compensate for feelings of inferiority. Others shop endlessly to deaden the pain. Some of us stuff our faces to avoid facing the truth. That was me. I spent a lifetime eating sugar, flour, and drive-through fast food to avoid experiencing feelings and situations that were uncomfortable.

Does this ever happen to you? Do you remember a time (or two) when you just didn't want to face it? Maybe a report that was due? Perhaps telling your favorite aunt that you couldn't attend her anniversary party? Letting your spouse know you got a speeding ticket? We avoid situations all the time. Some of us use food as the fallback answer—the answer to feeling alone, celebrating a reward, drowning out bad news of a job loss or a family tragedy. We stop using food as fuel for our bodies and begin using it as a drug, a process that often starts in childhood.

A Six-Year-Old Sugar Addict

When I think about my own addiction to sugar and flour, I first look to my parents to find the answers. My father was vastly over-weight, jolly, and affectionate. My mother, on the other hand, was (in my child eyes) underweight, serious, and strict.

At the time I didn't understand my mother's very traumatic child-hood. I look at her sweet childhood photos and can't believe that she was called "Fatso" by her own grandmother. My mother was tiny, and still is, yet was berated by her grandmother. It wasn't until later in my life that I understood why my mother pressed so hard for me to stay slim, lose weight, be active, and not eat so much. I'm sure she didn't want me to suffer the pain and humiliation she experienced from her own family. My mom's very frightening experience of living through World War II in Berlin, Germany, was a breeding ground for anxiety and fear for her.

Her family's home in Berlin was destroyed by bombing. My grandmother took my mother and the four other children by the hands and white-knuckled their escape over a swinging, temporary bridge. They jumped on crowded trains and walked great distances in extreme weather and war conditions to a tent camp for safety.

My mother knows hunger. She lived in a tent city for months and ate turnips and dandelion salad daily that had been foraged from the grasslands beyond the camp and made in a broken cooking pot over a makeshift, upside-down wrought-iron "grill" pulled from the street gutters. Later, when the Americans flew over Europe, they performed airdrops of food to the starving people below. Bags of sugar and flour flew down magically from the air, and for the first time in what seemed to be an eternity to my mother, she dug her hand straight into a bag of sugar and ate it.

I had never experienced hunger, yet I had that same way of behaving toward sugar and flour as my mother did when she dug her hand straight into the bags of sugar decades ago. I have, as my mother did, a ferocious drive to consume all things sweet. Perhaps in my childhood years, my mother allowed me to indulge in these goodies so that I would feel the comfort she didn't have as a child. To be honest, whether she let me have them or not, I found a way to get my hands on the contraband—no matter what.

The Doughnut Shop

I had a special sugar bond with my dad. Every Saturday I would wake up and get dressed immediately. By 6:30 AM, I had already watched my fill of Bugs Bunny and Roadrunner cartoons, and was prepared to hit the road with my dad. He had a lot of work responsibilities, even on the weekends. I accompanied him on his morning routines: the first stop was our local country club where my father managed the books. He had special keys to get into the club before it was open, and while he collected all the receipts and reports from the week gone by, I would settle in at the bar and pretend I had some customers. I would serve Coke or 7-Up and mix it up with a maraschino cherry. The customer was actually me, and one maraschino cherry always led me to consume the entire jar of cherries. I loved that place and all the sugar that came with it.

The next stop with Dad was to a local nursing home where he would check on a client. My father was appointed as trustee for aging folks who didn't have family in our hometown. We would stop in and Dad's client would typically offer me a freshly baked cookie from her vintage owl cookie jar. Our morning continued with another stop to the local feed mill to visit my uncle Jerry, one of Wisconsin's top-producing dairy farmers, then on to the newsstand to get a Saturday morning paper for Dad and penny candy for me, and finally to the local doughnut shop.

Each and every Saturday, I could have whatever I wanted at the bakery. Imagine, nose pressed to the glass counter, asking, "Can I have that one?" Yes. "Can I get that one?" Yes. I ordered to my heart's content, and so did Dad. When we were done gleefully selecting our sugar prizes, I was reminded that we best take a few things home for the rest of the family. To me, this was an afterthought. I wondered if our baker could package up my doughnuts separately so that I wouldn't have to share. Didn't want any mix-ups or confusion about what was mine. When it came to desserts and baked goods, I would carry this thinking around with me for the rest of my life.

Looking back, these memories were indeed sweet (to my taste buds and in my mind's eye), but as an adult, this memory also brings with it a very jolting realization: my father, a severe diabetic, was my sugar buddy. At that time I was too young to understand that what my father was doing was like committing involuntary suicide. You can't eat sugar like we did and manage your life with diabetes. If I had only known. If only he had taken care of himself in a healthier way. For him, it is a shame he died at the young age of fifty-seven. For me it was a shame I learned that no matter how sick you are, you don't need to take care of yourself. Sugar and flour took my dad to his grave—and I learned that was okay.

Taking an Advance on My Allowance to Buy Sugar

I remember getting an allowance from my father and taking my money and my very confident little self to town every Saturday— sometimes walking and sometimes with my bike—to buy two things at the local dime store in my hometown: a new Barbie doll outfit and a boatload of candy.

Each Saturday I found I was spending more money than I had, and it didn't seem to matter. There I was, standing in line, suffering anxiously with my carefully selected wax lips, candy cigarettes (Pall Mall), Slo Pokes, and jawbreakers, knowing I didn't have enough money to pay for them. If I were lucky and my ever-prepared sister Pat was with me, I would ask her yet again if I could borrow the money "just this one time"—again—or I would muster up the gumption to ask the dime store cashier to loan me the money until I could pay her back.

Many Saturdays, this same cashier would listen to my heartfelt dilemma—very serious in nature—as I would promise to run home and bring the money back within the hour. Was I such a pest that I wore people down? Did I have a flair with convincing others? Was I just plain ol' manipulative? No matter what, I would leave the dime store, consuming candy like there was no tomorrow, and then run all the way home—to ask my sweet dad for an advance on next week's allowance.

My First Organizing Obsession—
or Was It Hoarding?

Eating and organizing candy was my favorite covert pastime. And the most revered of holidays, Halloween, could never appear on the calendar fast enough. Before trick-or-treating, I set up an efficient assembly line in my bedroom where I would group, count, and then eat my candy. Costumes were not the important part of Halloween; it was the candy. While other kids were busily discussing and planning their artistic disguises for this devilish October night, I was assessing the neighborhood strategically to gain access to the best and most abundant candy givers. After a night of trick-or-treating, I knew to the last mini candy bar where I stashed my contraband to hide from my mother. My sister, who knew I always had a candy factory set up, always demanded her cut of the action. It was like handing over hush money to keep the goods secret.

What was worse? The need to organize or the need to hide candy like a squirrel burying its nuts in the snow? My father was thrilled at my capability to organize my stuff; he could see in me the next banker in the family. Who knew that sugar consumption and organizing would come to me at such an early age? No wonder the correlation has become so evidently clear for me and many of the clients with whom I work.

When I think about organizing my stuff during my childhood, I needed to do it for three reasons:

1. It made my mother happy.
2. It came naturally to me.
3. It helped me gain control of my environment and my fears.

Wrestlers, Buses, and Cheerleaders—Oh, My!

At the age of six, I distinctly remember one of my first frightening events. I was a miniature cheerleader on the high school cheerleading squad, and on the weekends I would go with the big girls and my older sister Chris on the school bus to a basketball game or wrestling match. The state wrestling tournament was happening in the far-off and very big city of Madison, Wisconsin (not that far, really, and not that big then). In my pint-size pleated skirt and oversized pom-poms, I cheered all day for our champion wrestlers. Later that night, we were instructed to board our bus home. With the "big girl" cheerleaders guiding me, we made it to the bus and settled in for the trip home.

I kept looking for my sister Chris and was very worried that the bus driver would leave without her. More high school teenagers boarded the bus, but Chris was nowhere in sight. My forty-five-pound self was shivering in fear—the bus driver and school chaperones were making "last call." I was in total fear and panic, and I burst out and ran down the bus aisle to announce, "We can't go—my sister isn't here. Please, please don't go without her!"

Through my tears, I was reassured that my sister was there and had boarded the other bus home. I needed to see this for myself, so the bus driver brought my sister over to my bus to prove that she was safe. The big-girl cheerleaders came to my rescue, and soon after, my feelings were soothed with an ice cream cone at the local A&W, where our bus stopped on the way home. Translation: Have fear? Eat food. I've been doing it that way all my life.

"I'll Make You Something Special"

During those years, even though I yearned to eat junk food, I could count on my mother to always prepare a very healthy meal for me and the entire family. Before the war raged in Berlin, my grandmother would always make what her children wanted at mealtime. String-bean stew, Hungarian goulash, and potato pancakes were just a few of her specialties. If Grandma Lucy was preparing a delectable dinner and my mom didn't like it, Grandma would prepare something else: cheese blintzes or a pancake—something quick and sweet. Mother loved her mother's cooking; it made her feel special.

Just as history repeats itself, if I didn't like what my mother was making for dinner, she would make me a special meal as well. The whole family was being served spaghetti and meat sauce and Dorothy didn't like it? Pass the buttered noodles for me, please, and keep the veggies on the other side of the table. I got to eat what I wanted, and I grew up believing that I was special. Problem is, I didn't just believe that concerning the food. I believed I should have special privileges all the time! Somehow, I created the idea that I was the exception to every rule.

If others had to stand in line for something, I would angle to find a way to move to the front of the line. If all the kids had finals in college, I would speak to the dean of the college to get a special test date to accommodate my schedule. If everyone at the office was expected to work overtime during tax season, I solicited my boss to see things my way as to why I shouldn't have to. If I could take all those incidents back, I would. But I can't. This personal exclusivity stayed with me until I came to terms with my food addiction. Lots of apologies and a great big humble pill was the only way to solve this one.

The Only Way to Shut Her Up
Is to Quarantine Her

One thing hit me fair and square and taught me that I couldn't always have my way. When I was thirteen years old, I was diagnosed with acute bacterial spinal meningitis. I was hospitalized and quarantined for a month, and my friends, family, and schoolmates all took penicillin to avoid catching this contagious bacterium. My parents nervously watched my white blood count and visited me daily. While I definitely remember the painful spinal taps, hourly blood tests, and days of sheer hospital boredom, the biggest memory was the gifts that people brought me.

Everyone back then knew my favorite candy bar was Forever Yours, a 1.76-ounce bar of dark chocolate on the outside with a mix of caramel and nougat on the inside. I received more than sixty of these get-well candy-bar gifts. I ate all of them, and though I was told I would never be able to be athletically active again, I was. That's all this developing teen needed to learn, and it was sort of like what I learned with Dad and his diabetes: when you're sick and hospitalized, you reward yourself with chocolate!

As I made my physical comeback, I continued to reward myself with chocolate, and new on the food scene were entire packages of cookies accompanied by cold Wisconsin milk. My brother, Edd, who had recently returned from Vietnam, was trying to reclaim his own life postwar.

He kept to himself and listened to Led Zeppelin, Deep Purple, and Jethro Tull by the hour with the aid of his oversized and clear-sounding earphones. Edd noticed me, however. While my parents were at work—Dad at the bank and Mom at the adorable town flower shop—Edd commented on how amazed he was that I slammed down another package of cookies, and he didn't even get one. He was sort of making a joke of it, yet it stands out strongly in my memory today. What was I doing? Home after school, eat a package of Chips Ahoy, and sit down for an elegant meal prepared by Mom. It didn't end there. My father discovered Ho Ho wrappers in the glove box in the car, and my mother picked up even more candy wrappers in my room. The observation and confiscation were not limited to my own family. My hometown had nearly 5,000 people in it, and I swear each and every resident was watching what I ate. In high school I was a celebrated varsity gymnast, and if a town local saw me at the drugstore having a malt at the counter with the other kids, my parents knew about it before I could say "Boo." I was gaining weight and something had to give! But what?

I Can't Be Fat—I'm an Athlete

The scales still tipped in my favor. I was a champion gymnast in the making and worked out between three and four hours a day. Youth had its benefits: I could eat all the sugar, candy, ice cream, and junk I wanted and still maintain a sporty physique. Though my mother spent hours coaching me on good health or negotiating with me to lose weight in exchange for a new back-to-school wardrobe, I ignored her.

Throughout high school, I lived and loved my life. I attended dances with boys, was voted into the prom court, vacationed with my best friend and her parents or mine, participated in the student council, and won state championships in track and gymnastics. I even became Miss Richland County—tiara, sash, parades, floats—such fame and fortune (as I saw it). I was basking in the popularity, and I was receiving the attention I so desperately required.

Stop the Bus—That's My Dad on the Side of the Road

Despite my letterman's jacket, the awards, medals, and all the accolades my hometown locals bestowed upon me, I had fear. I worried that if I was too good of a gymnast, my teammates wouldn't like me. I worried that my high school boyfriend might find someone better. I worried that I interpreted my homework assignments differently than everyone else. I was afraid of not being on time, getting lost while driving in a big city, and dropping the baton in our 400-meter relay race. You name it, I worried about it. I worried most about my father's failing health. Just as when I was a six-year-old cheerleader and thought the bus was leaving my older sister behind, I had a strangely similar experience with my dad.

I share this story to reinforce how much fear I carried as a child—and still do today, except I have a way to manage it. It was a very cold and blizzardy night, and my coaches and our gymnastics team were on the school bus heading back from a gymnastics meet in Spring Green, only thirty-five minutes from home. My dad drove separately in his bad-ass gold Cadillac to watch me. He, too, was on his way home.

My parents attended nearly every meet, game, match, concert, and event I was in; they gave their lives to support me. What was there possibly to be afraid of? And why eat over it? Well, you can ask that same question of someone who hoards too much stuff or someone who drinks to escape the pain. For me, it's fear, doubt, and insecurity. Because my father was a very sick man—he looked seventy-five when he was a mere fifty-five years old—I carried a foreboding feeling around me with much of the time. I checked on him many nights as he sat in his rocking chair unable to sleep. I would try to make him laugh as he held his head in his hands in exhaustion at the kitchen table after work each day. I would walk slowly when we were together so as not to embarrass my father because he could not walk fast anymore. When I would compete, I would watch and wait for him to arrive safely before I could settle myself and perform. With all this in the background, as we drove along the dark and snow-drifted highway, our bus passed my dad's Cadillac—broken down, with flashers blinking at the side of the road. My dad! Another moment of fear was frozen in time for me. I ran to the bus driver and yelled, "Stop the bus! Please! My dad is stuck on the side of the road."

By this time my dad was a very frail man, and true to form, I was in a panic about him. Thankfully, the driver stopped the bus, turned it around, and went back to pick up my dad. As Dad slowly boarded the bus loaded with giddy gymnasts screaming, "Hi, Mr. Breininger," my dad took a seat at the front on the bus. Safe. Warm. Relieved. We both sat quietly arm in arm the rest of the ride home. We shared a cookie I had packed in my gym bag. My fear was not gone, but my dad was here for now. I don't think I ever shared these very private fears with anyone in my family—not even my friends. Cookie or no cookie, I think I knew that my father's eating lifestyle would be the death of him, and it never occurred that it could happen to me too.

Trapped in the Dorm and Covered in Parking Tickets

When high school ended, so did my father's life and my quest for gymnastics or any other kind of stardom. Though I was offered a gymnastics scholarship to the Air Force Academy, I chose to attend the University of Wisconsin–Madison, a college that's not easy to get into. With a gymnastics walk-on scholarship and letters of recommendation that would blow the most cynical minds, I was accepted—and only sixty miles away from home. I convinced myself that all the stars in the universe, no matter how infinite, pointed in my direction. But after I arrived, the stars flamed out, littered around my feet.

While most middle-aged men enjoyed the prime of their lives, Dad left this world both physically and mentally drained at age fifty-seven. While his golf swing was powerful, his eating and drinking for a man with severe diabetes were equally as such. Would my dad's death be a wake-up call for me? Nope. Instead, I continued to emulate his charm and kindness with the community, while stuffing myself with the only numbing agent I could count on: food.

I could have saved years of agony as an adult if—beginning in college, if not before—I would have used the word *no*. No to the wrong relationships, no to stupid mistakes, no to jobs that were offered to me but weren't for me, no to the people who took advantage of my good nature. For all intents and purposes, the word *no* was like a four-letter word banned in our household. My dad could soothe and calm the nastiest customers at the bank where he worked. A gentleman to a fault, he only wanted to please. But that same overly kind, calming exterior led to his binge eating and diabetes. Little did he realize that by saying no, he could have extended his life and created genuine happiness. But now one of his surviving daughters also found that people pleasing was an instant claim to fame—yet for years a devastating circular pattern of food bingeing accompanied the people-pleasing behavior.

UW–Madison is a testing ground for some of the smartest and most competitive students in the world. An education here would have meant graduate school at any Ivy League school. What an American success story . . . a small-town girl propels herself into gymnastics, then attends a world-renowned university only to add another cream-of-the-crop institution to a stunning résumé! Only that's not what happened. After my dad died, I could not face school, let alone my own life. I left after two years and cycled through bouts of depression with the help of my favorite companion. (Do I need to even say what it is?)

Before making the decision to leave, I entered the deepest, darkest, and loneliest periods of my life. I was living in a jock dorm on campus and couldn't get a grip on my father's death. I didn't understand anything about death or grieving, and I found myself turning to food for comfort. Worse yet, I stopped going to class, broke up with my high school sweetheart, and began to miss gymnastics practice. I lived in the dark—drapes closed by day, isolated, and eating excessive amounts of dorm food and junk food. Tons of food and no exercise is a certain prescription for weight gain and depression.

The more you eat, the more you eat—and the less you do, the less you do. It was bad. I was now the proud owner of my dad's gold Cadillac, which was permanently parked in the street behind my dorm—collecting parking ticket after parking ticket on the windshield. I didn't care. I was drifting and didn't know how to ask for help. The only help I summoned came in the form of a pint from the freezer section.

It wasn't long before my grade reports caught up with me, the numbers on my bathroom scale soared to new heights, my ATM card ran out of cash, my coach called me into her office, and my car was booted and fined. That's what college looked like for me.

Shortly thereafter, I quit school, quit gymnastics, and stopped dating altogether. I was aimless and felt lost. I applied to be a flight attendant, I interviewed for sales jobs, and then did what most people do when the going gets tough: became a cashier at McDonald's. And really, what better place for a gal with a food addiction than the Golden Arches? Easy access to burgers, fries, ice cream, and cookies.

Pass Me the Steno Book, Sir

Somehow, my sister Pat sensed my despair. She suggested it would be good for me to attend a secretarial school in Boston. In the early 1980s, this particular private school—Katharine Gibbs—was known for its Marine-like precision, turning out executive secretaries to top-flight companies. I made the move and graduated at the top of my class within a year. I requested interviews with Donald Trump and Jack Welch (then CEO of General Electric), as well as would-be governors and presidential hopefuls.

Plump and professional, I donned my mandatory panty hose and stiff business suits (accessorized by blouses with bowties) to showcase my super shorthand skills, typing speeds of 100-plus words per minute, my magical ability to file alphabetically while standing upside down, and my ability to master the intricacies of introducing international delegations to my high-powered bosses-to-be.

My tour at Katie Gibbs Secretarial School gave me a sense of adulthood, and I quickly became known as the intense secretary everyone wanted to hire. Within months I was working for a self-made multimillionaire in the printing business and later for the dean of the College of Business at Northeastern University. But my thirst was not quenched with work. I started eating again and dieting again—up and down the scale I went.

The Mysterious Older Man

Enter the "older man." At age twenty-one, I was living and working in Manhattan, and through my job I met a man who was eighteen years my senior. He was handsome enough, seemed worldly, sought my untapped opinions, and acted my age (later I learned that was the problem). Our courtship was a thrill. Though I was completely overweight, Bob courted me like I was a slim Heidi Klum. Elegant meals out, dancing until the wee hours, fancy hotels, basketball games at Madison Square Garden, skiing at swanky mountain resorts. In fact, Bob ran a hotel in New England and flew me up from New York City regularly to see him. What a jet-setter! Considering myself a smart person, and not wanting to get caught in any weird workplace romance situation, I used my position to access Bob's personnel file. The file said he had *been* married.

Later, I questioned him about his marital status. "Bob, I want to be sure you are divorced. You are divorced, aren't you?" He answered yes. Hallelujah. What a relief! We were free to date. It was a year later when I learned Bob was indeed twice divorced, but that he had left out an important detail: he was *still married* to someone else. Food to the rescue!

The good news is that I got out of the relationship with Bob immediately. The bad news is that he ended his relationship and begged me to take him back—and I did. Months later, when Bob's divorce was finalized, we moved in together and eventually married. At this point, I began fighting bitterly with my mother. Months would pass without our speaking to each other, and moments of laughter and softness were rare. Blame-filled conversations, followed by defensive letters via snail mail, followed by muddled hearsay among family members created two decades of pain for my mom and me. She really didn't like or trust Bob (wonder why?), and her approach was a bit off the mark in terms of delicacy. Worse yet, the few times I did see my mom—once or twice a year—didn't give us enough mother/daughter time to talk about the obvious issues in a compassionate way.

Always seeking my mother's approval, yet rarely honoring or respecting her, we always fell into a vicious cycle and painful discussion about my weight. It was all she seemed to bring up. "How did you get so big? What are you doing? Are you unhappy? What's going on with you?" So many invasive questions. But looking back, she was right on all counts. Mom could see my situation and I could not—and would not—want to hear a word. I was combative and volatile. I raised my voice often in my own defense, hell-bent to show my mom a thing or two. You know how? I ate more. So there! En garde—take that!

I was unforgiving to my mom and to myself. Could my mother have refined her approach to one of compassion toward me? Absolutely. Could I have just once agreed with her and affirmed that maybe she was right? Without a doubt. In order to figure out my life and finally reduce my weight, I had to come to terms with my own relationships—not only with Bob but, more importantly, with my mother.

Back then, I just didn't have the maturity or desire to learn why my mom and I couldn't get along. Certainly she had my best interests at heart, but she was suffering from her own traumatic past, and neither of us had the capacity to sit with each other's pain and problems. Did it really take me forty years to understand how great my mom is? Yes, and I'll share how I did it later.

The Extra-Large TV Persona

My final chapter in "living life large" came as a result of my appearance on television. I was regularly appearing and seeing myself on the *Dr. Phil* show as a life coach; on QVC with sellout segments for *Cherished Memories* (an interview book created by my business partners, Debby Bitticks and Lynn Benson; more on this later); on the *Today* show, the *Bonnie Hunt* show, *The View*, and *Nightline*; and on the PBS pledge show for another one of our company's products, *Our Life's Essential Information*. It was hard enough to watch myself on the taped segments of these shows, but the PBS show was set to re-air and re-air and re-air. Never before did I love the quality of the product so much and detest how I looked delivering the information. Night after night, I would flip the channel and cringe at how large I had become.

I also saw myself living life large on *Hoarders*. It was airing most Monday nights with millions of viewers, and when I was watching myself work with people who hoarded too much stuff, I suffered with my own underlying truth: I was hoarding, too—on my hips, tummy, in my neck (what sleep apnea? what snoring?), everywhere.

Though I had begun gaining insight about myself over the years while filming *Hoarders*, it finally dawned on me like the startled "surprise" that horses exhibit at the racetrack when they are released from the gates: I needed to do something for myself—not for anyone else, but just for me.

If I wanted to really step into my powerful self and help others, and have them know they could count on me not just for what I said but for what I did, I needed to change. I researched sugar addiction, which led me to study food addiction—and then I *finally* jumped in with no turning back. My life has never been, nor will it ever be, the same. Seventy-five pounds lighter for me meant a healthy dating relationship, a solid community around me, being nice to my mom, apologizing quickly when I was wrong, being on time, returning phone calls, climbing stairs without wheezing, sleeping solidly through the night, increased business, more money in my bank account, and more time to enjoy my life.

I stopped stuffing my face and started facing my stuff, one area
of life at a time. In the following chapters you will read about my
"befores and afters," learn some of the information I used to make
the change, and see how I saw correlated clutter and hoarding to
weight loss—and you'll get a few tips to start off in the right direction, too.

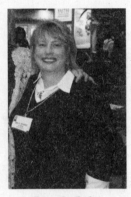

Dorothy Before

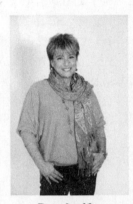

Dorothy After

I tell you my life story as my way of demonstrating to you that I
have truly experienced every chapter of this book—whether finances
or failures, the state of being overwhelmed (with emotions or situations), or lack of self-esteem. I have without a doubt stuffed my
face to avoid facing my stuff. The coming chapters are meant to give
you a leg up, a quicker path, or an enlightened approach to facing
down the stuff you've been avoiding. Once you tackle the first area
of life that is plugging the dam, the rest will release for you. Whether
it's too much clutter, too many pounds, overworking, or drinking
in excess, the following chapters will assist you in fighting for your
health, family, and life.

2

FACING IT:
Do You Have a
Food Obsession?

As you can see, my experiences on *Hoarders* taught me a lot. Yes, my role on the show is as the "expert organizer," but in shedding excess weight, I can now see so many similarities between my overweight self and the folks who hoard. There were clues everywhere in my life that pointed to why I was overweight: candy wrappers in the car, voice mail that was full from not returning phone calls in a timely fashion, overspending on my food budget, and a bulging closet of clothes—because I kept buying the next size up and the next size up.

In terms of clutter, the more stuff that appears on our desks, in our cars, in our homes, on our already-crowded calendars, and on our bodies just might be clues to something else going on in our lives—something that we might not be facing.

Pink Passion

Denise was a sweet, petite, hardworking mother of five. She collected clothing, bought clothing, shopped for clothing, borrowed clothing, kept clothing, and hoarded clothing, and a few other things, too. Denise's home, though filled primarily with boys, was chock-full of her feminine frippery, her pretty clothing, her stuff. No matter what the family said, she couldn't really see it as a hoarding home, although all the clues were there.

When people walked into Denise's home, they would battle just to open the front door. Once inside, you could follow a path strewn with chest-high glittery dresses, purses made of pink faux fur, purple fishing tackle–like boxes overrun with sparkling costume jewelry, and over-the-top hair clips. This man-made Wall of China in the living room guided you like a maze to either the kitchen or a dangerously packed staircase that led to the family bedrooms. In the kitchen, the dishwasher served as a filing cabinet for kids' report cards from school, lab tests from the doctor, and holiday cards from years gone by.

The clutter was speaking loud and clear! Do you know what the clutter was really saying? (Yeah, if only clutter could talk.) The clutter was a physical manifestation of what Denise wanted to say: "I don't like my marriage and I don't like how I'm being treated by my family anymore." There was only one solution: face her stuff! First, she had to clear out the physical mounds of excess dresses, purses, shoes, toys, and jewelry. Second, she had to face her marriage and her family. The wall of stuff could no longer be the dividing line between Denise and all of her relationship issues. She needed to speak up.

Just as my candy wrappers and stacked-up restaurant receipts were clues to my own obesity, it was the same for Denise and her obsession with clothes. *Hoarders* cast a glaring, squinting,

I-can-hardly-see kind of light on Denise and her clutter. It leveled her, and she broke down in tears. She finally gained the self-awareness she needed in order to turn the corner and begin practicing self-control in the future.

Just like Denise, spotlights were flashing on me, too (I wore sunglasses most of the time and ignored the flashing lights); however, I also had a turning point. I finally paid attention to the physical clues and my mind clutter to determine how to clean up my act.

What does your clutter or disorganization say about you? Though you may not be experiencing a massive hoard, that unopened pile of bills on the kitchen counter may just be the suggestion you can use to identify areas of dissatisfaction that are leading you to continued weight gain, overspending, gambling, or some other addictive behavior.

I finally understood wholly what my friend and colleague Peter Walsh was writing about in his book, *Does This Clutter Make My Butt Look Fat?* I witnessed the struggle that each of my hoarding clients endured to stop their wicked behavior, whether it was picking up usable stuff from the side of the road or whisking an entire shelf's worth of sale items into their shopping carts to take home, only to leave the bags gently stacked on top of more unopened bags from Walmart or Goodwill.

I couldn't stop my insatiable overeating behavior either. Each day on the *Hoarders* set, I would work calmly and lovingly with an individual who hoarded, and at night I went back to the hotel and ate. Where was the calm and loving compassion for myself? Why was it so easy to give to others and not be able to summon that compassion up for myself?

Often, I would cry after leaving the set location, usually on the plane ride home. Sometimes it was because the hoarding family on the show had such tragic circumstances, and sometimes it was because I had my own. My colleagues on the show—the producers, camera and sound people, the other experts—watched and noticed my unwillingness to share my story and my life. I'm sorry for that. I could have used their support and just didn't know how to ask for it, much like the individuals on *Hoarders*. They just didn't know how, and someone (my colleagues and I) had to show them the way. I had to find my way, too. I honestly believe that I released my own body clutter because of the episodes I filmed for *Hoarders*. My hoarding clients taught me this lesson—and all the while I was thinking *I* was the expert on the show! (How about some humble pie now, Dorothy?)

As for Denise and her obsession with clothes, in addition to not wanting to face her relationships, she had lost sight of her goals and dreams. Denise's clutter reflected her unhappiness. What does *your* clutter say about you? Are you consistent with your goals and dreams? Do your actions support your goals and dreams? Does the stuff around you enhance your goals and dreams? If not, the time has come to reacquaint yourself with those goals and dreams and learn how you can make small changes to get closer to them.

Let Your Goals Guide You:
Goal Setting Inspires and Keeps You Honest

My goals and dreams saved my life. In my late twenties I was ready to pursue a lifelong dream. Traveling was flowing in my veins. I do not mean the two-week vacation in a cabin by a lake and boat rides for tourists. I mean a one-year vacation around the world with my best friend, Donna, complete with one backpack per person and a spending limit of $5,000 each for the entire year, including all flights, trains, boats, and even camel transportation! We planned this for fourteen months, and just by declaring this dream to the world, I soon discovered that I was taking better care of myself. Yes, the power of goals and dreams! In an instant, junk food and excess portions meant little to me. I was back in the saddle again, planning and loving life to the hilt.

Bob was not interested in traveling whatsoever, yet he encouraged me to seek my dream. I could not have asked for a more practical person as a traveling companion than Donna. We are both from the Midwest, and we made fast friends at Katherine Gibbs Secretarial School. Donna also graduated at the top of our class and paid her way through an Ivy League school, receiving a degree in archaeology. We complemented each other with our skill sets. I was the perfectly organized person, detailing each item to go into our backpacks. I knew the timetable of all the flights, trains, buses, and boats. This was my calling, and I *loved* the passion I felt when doing this. At times, Donna and I seemed to be polar opposites, and thankfully she knew how to pitch a tent, figure out what to take when staying at a hostel in the Arctic, or how to stretch our budget right down to the shilling, pound, and deutsche mark.

From the very beginning of the trip, with my own minimalist packing, and then throughout our travels to Cairo, the Australian outback, and Leningrad, I rapidly noticed that from region to region, people owned less, bought less, and seemed happier with less stuff. The farther we traveled from the over-advertised, media-saturated cities, people seemed to be lighter, full of smiles, and extremely helpful. This trip was the classroom education I needed to start a new business in organizing and helping others decide what they valued most.

With just one key on my key chain and no phones to answer, I visited new friends' homes around the world, and in almost every case, people in foreign lands had very little clutter in their homes. I had the opportunity to see firsthand in Russia how families merged together—three generations sometimes, all in one very small apartment. In Thailand, entire families lived on floating rafts the size of my modest dining room, and in Egypt, during my bike ride through the countryside, folks lived in mud huts with no doors or windows—wide open for me and everyone else to peer into. And there wasn't much stuff in there.

I interviewed individuals across thirty-three countries and learned firsthand that the fewer items they had, the fewer decisions they had to make, the less they had to buy, and the less money it took for them to feel successful, which allowed for more time with family and friends. I learned about more than just geography, culture, art, and people. I learned values. Traveling with less, not having the space in my pack to purchase items, and being away from my home—free of all my possessions—taught me to enjoy the few things I had and focus more on myself and the people with whom I was visiting. And isn't it interesting that by focusing on my own life dreams, my own self-care, and others' needs, I dramatically shed fifty pounds?

Of equal interest, traveling with Donna was like having a private museum docent by my side. We ran the Olympic track in Greece wearing handmade olive branch crowns. We visited Topkapi Palace Museum in Turkey, where all the married men wanted to show us around. Donna had already studied the paintings we were now seeing in person: Dali's work at Prado in Spain, Degas' work in Paris's Musée de l'Orangerie, and the Rosetta Stone in the National Museum in London. She was brilliant and became my teacher of all things I had missed in my own high school and college education.

One particular memory will keep Donna in my mind forever. Though I was born and raised in a small town, my upbringing was rather metropolitan. I had never camped or used a compass in my entire life up to that point; I relied on Donna's "orienteering" days from her youth. We had taken a train to Zermatt, Switzerland—snowy winter lands surrounding us, with the stunning Matterhorn in the distance. The weather was unreasonable, yet it was our once-in-a-lifetime chance to hike the Swiss Alps. Always determined and prepared, Donna set the course.

We left promptly at 10:00 AM with a flashlight, emergency sleeping bags, waterproof matches, rain gear, and a hand-drawn map. We knew to expect a two-and-a-half-hour climb, but the fog, rain, and snow on the ground increased our foot travel time up the mountain to four hours. Prior to leaving, we checked in at the base camp to let others know where we were going and what time we left. On our way to the trailhead, we stopped to honor the hundreds of mountaineers who had lost their lives tackling these dangerously alluring mountains. It frightened me, but Donna was undaunted.

Farther along, we passed through small villages built into the side of the mountain—frozen laundry hanging on the clothesline, snowdrifts blocking the front door of these meager mountain dwellings. We got up high enough and started hiking the switchbacks in the thick, misty fog. Up and up and up we trekked until we reached the thick, snow-laden trails, with earlier hikers' footprints still visible. We truly hoped the sun would poke through, but it continued to get cooler. I put on my turtleneck, scarf, and gloves as it began to snow. We periodically stopped to assess our situation: Too much fog? Proper shoes? Steepness of trail? How soon before it gets dark? Recheck all of our supplies. No one else around? Material to mark the trails? Were we crazy or just adventurous?

Just as we made our very safe, mature decision to turn around, the sun pressed through the clouds. We could see we were near a monumental vista point to view the Matterhorn in its glory. We took it as a sign and gave ourselves one more hour to march forward. We promised ourselves—no matter what—that we would turn around at 2:00 PM.

At 1:45 PM we knew it was nearly time to turn around. Disappointed, but always optimistic, Donna sang her usual "Sunshine on My Shoulders" by John Denver. I rolled my eyes. She laughed. The sun miraculously appeared. *Wahoo! Yes, I can see the Matterhorn! Oh my Lord, what a view!* Filled with jubilation, I ran to the side of the trail to grab a shot of this mammoth mountain peak. The sun was creating a bizarre daytime light show, one to only rival the aurora borealis. Diamond prisms formed on winter plants, raindrops frozen in time, reflected like fancy French chandeliers. As we stood there, we were greeted by dense fog, alternating with bright sunshine and crisp clear views. It was wild. If ever I were looking for a spiritual connection, this was the day.

And then it happened, the one experience you wait your entire life for. You never know when it's going to happen, and you don't even know what "it" is. My turn was now. It was 2:30 PM, time to descend the mountain. Just as we turned to leave, the wind stopped and the sun commanded the mountaintops only. Donna screamed! Across the mountaintop next to us was a circular rainbow. A full circle rainbow! It was unbelievable. Fumbling for our cameras, we went to snap a shot of this mysterious event and noticed something even more remarkable; our shadows were cast onto the other mountain and we were *inside* that rainbow. I was silenced. I was inspired. I was quiet. I was fulfilled.

The sun took hold and guided us down the summit, lighting our path fully the whole way home. We had discovered the beauty we missed on the way up, which had been shrouded in the morning fog. Upon arrival, my thighs were tight, my ears were chilled, and my feet were wet from the deep snow at higher elevations. I had just experienced my first miracle. Little did I know there was another miracle right around the corner.

As Donna and I continued our journey beyond Switzerland to watch precision figure skaters in St. Petersburg in Russia, ride camels in Egypt's Sahara Desert, and meet up with and stay at the home of Czechoslovakia's premier swimming coaches, I noticed my clothes were too big. My shoes no longer fit my feet, my dress seemed two sizes too large, and my pants kept falling down! No way! Really? Had I lost weight?

I hadn't looked in mirrors that much because I was preoccupied with life. It seemed like overnight, I took a magic potion and *kaboom*! My body was its normal size! How could this be? Donna and I decided to go to every continent and enjoy the native food of each culture; whether buying it at an outside market or eating our packed picnics on a train, we experienced ethnic food that could only be savored in each country. Can you imagine drinking Russian vodka from a vending machine outside the Hermitage Museum, home of the czars? Yes, at times I ate the rich finger cakes served in European coffeehouses, but this time it was not to drown out my misery, but to inhale the flavors of each culture. I came home in perfect physical health, with clear skin and glossy hair. I had found the much-vaunted balance of life. For a fraction of time, I felt exhilarated. Indeed, that was also a miracle and one of my biggest life lessons—all because I declared a goal and shared my dream.

Your Goals and Dreams: New Thinking for Weight Loss

Somewhere back in my candy bar haze, I got the whack-a-doodle idea that "fun" was no longer for me. Have you lost any of your exhilaration for life? I somehow figured I didn't deserve it, nor did I have the energy to follow through with fun plans when I did make them. Now that I am free and clear of sugar and flour, I am reclaiming my childlike wonder and curiosity, and I'm relearning how to have fun without focusing on the food. My urge to have fun is being propagated. I can see that silliness and laughter improve my mental health.

Do you need more laughter and fun? If you do, make the move to enjoy your life and re-create your goals and dreams. You will find that because you're satisfying that missing piece in your life, suddenly you become more responsible about your finances, home, personal growth, and education—all of which improves your mental health, which in turn eliminates the cravings for food or other addictions. That is why when I work on my goals, I include the big and the small, the serious and the silly. If you wish to take a look at what you need or want to accomplish over the next year or the rest of this year, you can start right now. It doesn't matter if it's November and the year is almost over; the time to think about your goals is now. Here is a list of nine goal-oriented questions that I've created for you. Remember: those of you who actually take just a few moments to jot down some answers (any answers) have an increased chance of making your dreams come true and shifting your life. Go on, grab a pen.

1. List two things you can do to improve your health or fitness in the coming year:

   _____

   _____

2. List two recreational activities you might want to try in the coming year:

   _____

   _____

3. Educationally, do you have an interest to learn anything new? If so, list it here:

   _____

   _____

4. Regarding family and friends, does anyone need a little more attention from you? Do you feel the need to contact a long-lost friend? Do you need to practice saying no a little more to someone? Do you want to increase time with someone you really enjoy being around or maybe even decrease contact with someone who is a bit toxic?

   _____

_____

_____

_____

5. Do you need anything in your wardrobe, or do you want to get rid of anything?

_____

_____

6. If you are currently working, what would you like to change about your physical environment, or perhaps your own attitude?

_____

_____

7. Does your house/apartment/condo need repair? Do you need to purchase something? Need to get rid of anything? List a couple of goals to support your living environment.

_____

_____

8. Do you want more spirituality in your life? Want to learn about it? What would make you feel more spiritual?

_____

_____

9. Are you overspending in any area? Do you need to start a new savings account? Have you thought about talking to a financial planner?

_____

_____

Now, if you're looking for a less-structured approach to designing your goals and dreams, creating your own list of answers to the following questions might help. I've started you off with five examples in each section.

What are ten things I want to do in my lifetime?

1. Take golf lessons
2. Host a family art show
3. Whiten my teeth
4. Try ballroom dancing
5. Plan a weekend bike trip and stay at bed-and-breakfasts
6. _____
7. _____
8. _____
9. _____
10. _____

What are ten things I want?

1. To live on the ocean
2. To be married again to a very loving man
3. A combination of a feminine and athletic wardrobe
4. A massage every other week
5. A puppy
6. _____
7. _____
8. _____
9. _____
10. _____

What are ten fantasy experiences I would like to have?

1. Attend an exclusive ball
2. Stay in the best hotel in the world
3. Take a dream analysis class
4. Ride on a private plane
5. Have an amazing vintage flower garden
6. _____

7. _____

8. _____

9. _____

10. _____

How Goal Setting Can Get You Back to Your Ideal-Size Body

When it comes to being overweight, I've always held this silly thought in my head that the less you do, the less you do, and the more you do, the more you do. Perhaps I got this from my mom, who never stops moving—ever! Or perhaps it's a learned behavior. When I have goals and dreams written down with specific tasks to get there, I am more apt to do them. Once in motion, I stay in motion. When I was into food, I was far less active and less motivated overall.

While I was always reaching for my dreams, I encountered moments when the less I did (watch TV, eat, nap), the less I wanted to do, and that kept me sedate, which kept the calories collecting, which made me gain more weight, which kept me from getting involved. Watch the progression of how—for one of my clients—creating just one small goal and sharing it with someone can change your life:

✓ You want to go horseback riding, but you say, "I'm too overweight."

✓ Set a goal. Write it down: "I want to go horseback riding."

✓ You flip through a magazine at the dentist's office the next day and see an article on horseback riding. Ask the receptionist if she would photocopy the page for you; they usually appreciate that.

✓ Tape article on bathroom mirror. Smile.

✓ Surfing through the channels to find your favorite program
   a couple of nights later, you see a PBS show on the gypsy
   horse. You watch it instead. You learn that this horse and
   other draft horses can accommodate heavier riders. Maybe it
   is possible to ride.

✓ Over the weekend, you are out shopping and see adorable
   note cards with horses on them. You buy them. Later in
   the weekend, you actually send a note to a friend using the
   new note card and mention to your friend how you've been
   thinking of riding horses, how you would love to do it but
   have concerns about your weight. You wish your friend well
   and mail the card.

✓ A week later your friend calls you and tells you about a horse
   show that's coming to the area and thought you might like
   to go watch and just pet the horses in the stalls. You kind of
   question the coincidence of it all and say yes.

✓ The following weekend, you are out and about, moving
   your body, and enjoying the horse show. You're feeling more
   engaged in the world, and you're doing something in which
   you're interested. Life is good. Happy endorphins are moving
   around in your brain. You're breathing clean, healthful air.
   You pick up some brochures at the horse show and learn
   that, in four months, a nearby equestrian center is offering
   riding lessons. You take the brochure home and post it on the
   bathroom mirror.

✓ With the possibility in sight, you start taking the stairs each
   day at work rather than the elevator, and you notice you're
   down just a couple of pounds in a week and a half. How
   could it be that easy? Some evenings, you click onto the
   equestrian center's website to see if the riding classes are still
   offered. They are. The phone rings, and it's your sister-in-law.

You tell her about this string of coincidences regarding the horses and ask her opinion about signing up for the class. She supports your idea with excitement.

✓ The next day, on your way home from work, you swing by a discount clothing store to pick up a new pair of tennis shoes. The store has a new shipment of cowboy boots and has a pair in your size. Is it coincidence? Perhaps. Is it the effects of writing down a goal and sharing it? Definitely. Knowing you can return the boots, you buy them and place them prominently in your bedroom so that you see them each morning. You kind of feel motivated and decide it really may be possible for you to ride horses again. You decide to walk for ten minutes each evening before dinner.

✓ Between walking the stairs at work for a few weeks and walking before dinner during the last week (which has you less hungry at dinner), you can actually feel like you're losing some weight. It inspires you. You eat just a little less at dinner and cut out the 2:00 PM candy bar. Less sugar and flour in the day allows for a better night's sleep, and suddenly that old eating pattern shifts. Better sleep, less sugar, more walks, more stairs, more good endorphins, and a goal with people to talk to about it and events to attend. It seems almost certain you should sign up for riding lessons.

✓ So you do. You sign up. The minute you sign up, a sense of satisfaction floods you and suddenly, the more you do, the more you do. You are more social and talking to more people about your new, upcoming class, and you're feeling slimmer as the months go by. You go dancing at a nightclub on Friday night and hiking on Sunday. Your goal begins to permeate all aspects of your life. Eventually the horseback riding class begins and you enjoy it for an entire semester, which leads to another class, and you make new friends who are like-minded. A singles equestrian trip to Costa Rica is now on the horizon, and a few coffee dates, too.

Is it possible? Oh yes, just the single act of having my client write down a goal and share it with friends had her achieve a lifelong dream of riding horses. Writing down a goal and having a dream come true can happen for any of us: horses, skydiving, going to night school, changing jobs, traveling the world, or losing thirteen pounds. What's your goal? At the end of this book, you will be encouraged to create your own action plan. Write it down. Share it. Watch your life change. Watch your health change.

My own goal to travel the world taught me that I wanted to continue on an intermittent basis to insert some big, bold life dreams into my "regular" life. When it came to work, I was responsible, accountable, and dependable, yet I knew I needed to intersperse those traditional ways of living with the outrageous, the adventurous, and the spectacular. I saw my own father pass away before he had a chance to enjoy the fruits of his very hard labor, and I refused to make that same mistake. I knew I had to work to make a living, and I knew intuitively that I had just one life on this planet and I had to make the most of it.

I had a fire in my belly. I wanted more. I confided in my super knowledgeable and solution-oriented friend Nancy. I told her that I was proud of my world travel accomplishment and that people began to notice me—not for how I looked or even what I said, but for what I was up to in my life. Nancy encouraged me to pursue my dreams. For the last twenty-two years, Nancy has been my sounding board for new ideas and goals. She didn't steer me wrong then, and she never steers me wrong now. When I returned from my around-the-world tour, colleagues began asking me how they could take such a trip. They told me, "Oh, Dorothy, you're so lucky; you got to travel the world."

"No! This was not luck!" I would tell them. This was a dream, a written goal, a focused desire. In addition to writing down the goal, "I want to travel the world," I wrote down the thirty-seven steps I needed to take in order to create the trip of my dreams. I told my friends and colleagues they could do the same. If you want to go back to school, get a divorce, get married, travel the world, sell your home, adopt a child, or get your black belt in martial arts, you can do it! You have to state the goal, write down the steps, and begin to take action.

In addition to my travel goal, I knew I wanted to eventually own my own company. I read about successful CEOs who would take a private retreat for a week or two to redesign their companies. My year abroad was a retreat of sorts, and I began looking at what I loved to do plus what I was good at doing. I noticed a few things. (1) Because I had a lifetime of experience as an executive assistant to deans, chancellors, and CEOs, I was adept at managing other people's needs efficiently and effectively. (2) I observed myself seeing patterns and groupings of "like" things in such ways that others wanted to experience what I had to offer. (3) My thinking was a bit unique and unusual, which was inspiring for others and for me. During that trip I was able to transform my nonconforming, obsessive color coding and off-the-beaten-path kind of thinking into a profitable business—from secretary to entrepreneur.

I sketched ideas, journaled my thoughts, and made decisions to pare down my own life's possessions to support my dream. I knew then that the fewer items I was acquiring, dusting, packing, moving, and lugging around in life would free up my energy and time to create the business of my dreams, which would fit my personality and lifestyle to a T. I also discovered that as I took these steps for myself, I wanted to help others break free from the shackles we call "stuff."

Upon my return from my trip around the world, the name of my company—the Center for Organization and Goal Planning—was born, and what better place to launch it than Beverly Hills, where people have a lot of stuff and money to spend? While Bob preferred routine, he was enthusiastic and supportive of my new business idea and jumped at the chance to move from Boston to California to shake up our lives.

The Dirty Little Secret

My dear client—and now friend—Dee Dee Wilson Barton has a dirty little secret. She is a mother who is in a state of perpetual shock because she just didn't expect motherhood to be so hard! She is a chick with a potty mouth; she loves martinis, parties, and kids who are quiet. She also called me in a panic over paperwork not long after I started my business in California, and instead of just managing her paperwork, we discussed her life goals—and her life changed. Author of the book *The Dee View*, she writes,

I love those daytime talk shows. You know, *Dr. Phil* and *Kelly & Michael*. Nothing too *Jerry Springer*, but you get the idea. Anyhow, I was listening to *Dr. Phil* and tidying up my house when I heard about this professional organizer. And she was organizing a house in our neighborhood. I stopped cleaning and picking up toys (which my heart wasn't really into anyway), and I sat down. There was this adorable, professional blond woman: Dorothy Breininger, professional organizer. She radiated competence, and I needed some!

What caught my attention was *not* that she was cleaning up a hoarding house (have I mentioned "tidying" and "picking up" and "cleaning" yet? I love an organized house). She was talking about principles of organization. My husband and I own an accounting firm. At the time we were *drowning* in paperwork. (This was before scanners were ubiquitous. Dorothy and I were much younger then!) Some of our clients' data had slipped through the cracks, and we had missed a couple of deadlines for people. We took such pride (hey, we still do!) in giving great service and taking excellent care of our customers.

So I hit the Record button on the DVR, and that night, I made Greg watch this "Dorothy" girl. I told him, "I think she has the ability to really help our business." Who knew that was the *understatement* of the decade! Now just a bit about me: Do *not* stand in my way when I am on a mission. I tracked Dorothy—okay, I stalked her a little bit—and told her what I needed. I asked her to [gulp] come to our then-office in Palmdale, California. It turned out that tweaking our business systems to be more efficient and error-free was easy for Dorothy.

But what really changed our lives? She asked us a question—a simple, little question: "Is this business exactly where you'd like it to be?" Well, it covers most of our bills, but it would be great if we could grow it. A little more profit would be awesome. And it would be truly wonderful if we could find some really amazing staff. (Hiring the right team was a bumpy one "back in the day.")

Follow-up question: "Where would you like to be living eventually?" (Not that Palmdale wasn't the place to live out one's dreams.) Oh, well, we can't leave Palmdale. Our business that we built from nothing is here. My mama is here and she has dementia, and we take care of her. And she's in pretty good health, except for the dementia, so we can't leave; my relatives live well into their nineties. We are here for at least ten more years. Besides, uh, the cost of living is good. And did I mention that we built this business from nothing? The Yellow Pages and a phone. Yup, that was how we got started.

Question 3: "Do you want to live in Palmdale forever?" No! "Where would you like to live?" My husband and I looked at each other and responded together, "Palm Springs." So Dorothy wanted us to talk about Palm Springs. My response: "But it makes me uncomfortable 'cause of my mama." But we talk anyway. We were paying Dorothy to help us live a better life, so we might as well answer her silly questions.

(It just so happens that we had already done a demographic analysis, Palm Springs being our favorite vacation spot.)

Dorothy makes us really develop a business transition plan (against our will—there was kicking and screaming). What would we do with our Palmdale office? How would we develop a new business in Palm Springs? How would we go about marketing and hiring? During this period of our lives, I kept wailing, "This is a waste of time!" But it was so fun. So we kept working with Dorothy. We learned how to upgrade the quality of our staff. We practiced how to motivate the excellent team we had built and made them better. We didn't miss deadlines or lose paper. Okay, almost. And our business started growing. Our referrals went way up. The bottom line started looking better and better. And then my beloved mother passed away, quite suddenly.

After a few months, to get through the loss and life changes and get back on our feet, we were miraculously ready. And by "ready," I mean, there was nothing to it because during our vision and planning work with Dorothy, we had already made a detailed plan. We were going to move to Palm Springs! We had professional home staging done, and it made our lovely but lived-in home look like a model house. (Yes, we rented a storage pod and sifted through tons of toys.) And how about this? A full-price offer *the first day*!

We dropped 100 letters to all accounting firms in Palm Springs asking if anyone was interested in selling their firm, creative terms to be worked out. (Fingers crossed, candles lit—*Aummm*.) We found a house in Palm Springs (our poor real estate agent—three big dogs, two little kids, trekking from house to house), and an office in downtown and an office manager. *Boom, boom, boom.* Within a year, we had moved to Palm Springs and set up our second accounting office. Within two years we had tripled our business revenue. Two years after that we were even larger. Now we serve 1,300 clients, and our revenue is more than we ever imagined.

Let me be clear—we work hard in our business. It is called "work" for a reason. (There are no kayaks or lakes at our office!) But I am proud of the firm we have built—our super-professional and lovely staff—our efficiency and the great level of service we provide. And just in case you think there was a magic wand that Dorothy waved, let me clarify that as well. We do annual retreats with Dorothy and our team. We do business planning sessions with Dorothy twice a year. We even started doing personal goals and strategy development with Dorothy. We use her services for hiring and firing decisions. And we grow. And we become more proficient.

We always review and create goals and dreams. This process allows me to design my life each and every year in a way that serves me and my family and those around us, too.

Whether you do it by yourself or with your spouse, sibling, friend, or a professional, it's not *who* you do the goal planning and life dreaming with, it's *that* you do it all! In order to achieve your goals when it comes to weight loss, I have identified the top saboteurs that derail many of my clients. Once you tackle this clutter in your life— both mental and physical—it is much easier to be healthy.

Face Your Food Obsession

Does any of this sound familiar to you?

- One bite leads to another bite.
- One drink leads to another drink.
- One purchase leads to another purchase.
- One extramarital affair leads to another.
- One bet at the track leads to another.
- One shove or hit leads to another.
- One cigarette leads to another.

Don't be ridiculous! Food obsession? Me? Not possible! Won't say it. Don't believe it. Nonsense. I don't have an obsession. It's like saying I'm an alcoholic with food. It's like saying, "I can't stop even when I know eating certain foods and quantities are bad for me." It's like saying, "I'm always looking for the next hit, except it's with sugar." I refuse! I refuse! There is nothing wrong with me; it's just a food problem. I don't have the willpower. It's just that I can't stop eating certain foods even though my intellectual self knows better. True, it's sort of like I'm always looking for the next hit, but a food addict? Well, maybe. Let's take a look.

I really don't want to talk about this. I'm just too embarrassed. I would rather lie. I understand that's what many addicts do: Lie. Lie about how they may have gambled away the rent money. Lie about the $600 pair of boots they just had to have (which are hidden in the closet upstairs). Lie about consuming another bottle of odorless vodka carried secretly at the bottom of a suitcase when traveling.

Those addictions weren't mine. Mine was food, and I'm not that person anymore. I am no longer someone who has to lie about her food. I just didn't want you to know what I was eating back then, as if you couldn't guess I was sneaking something somewhere; it was kind of obvious if you took a look at me. Polite as I might be at a dinner out with colleagues and clients, ordering a proper salad and declining dessert, you can be sure I was having a private party in my very own kitchen every night once the formalities were over.

I cringe at the money I spent on my emotional and addictive eating. I squirm at the unending battle in my head not to go back to the fridge for the other pint or bag of whatever. I cower in the face of my roommates, boyfriends, sisters, mother, and friends who gently hid the expensive boxes of candy from me, and my hyper-sensing ability to match any crime scene investigator to find that box and shake it down until there was nothing left—except more embarrassment about where the stuff had gone come morning. Every night it seemed like I consumed the contents of an entire 7-Eleven, and every morning I swore it would never happen again—just like an alcoholic promises that "this time" it's his or her last bender.

My benders and binges always started at the grocery store. Shopping for the week ahead, I would purchase all the items from the middle aisles in the store—you know, the processed foods section: chips, cookies, boxed rice meals, mac and cheese. I would move to the freezer aisle for ice cream, frozen treats, and a bit of lighter fare (Popsicles), followed by a long layover in the bakery section, where I would pick up entire cakes and delicacy platters of petit fours, cupcakes, and mini-pastries—for a party I was attending, I would tell the cashier—but really just for me.

I still don't want to tell you this, but I'll continue, because sharing is what we do when we're recovering from an addiction, and I've got plenty to share. Following my insane food shopping event, I would begin consuming a mix of sugary bits and salty treats while driving the short distance to my home. Hungry or not, I could not even imagine waiting the ten minutes to get home and eat. Ahhhh, but you see, there was another quick side trip to make. Perhaps a swift drive-through at the fast-food joint to pick up a magic iced coffee jacked with flavoring, sugar, and whipped cream to sip. I'm horrified, but I was so craving-crazed to get to the drive-through window, I could have driven over all the other cars waiting in line to pick up their own Happy Meals. Hurry up! Move out of my way, for goodness sake.

Once home, my groceries did not make it out of all the bags immediately. I unpacked just enough of the groceries to get to the treasures buried within. Once I found the cold milk and package of cookies, I would sit in front of my big-box TV and begin eating in synchronization with the scripted actors on the screen (while watching the clock because I had a dinner engagement in two hours). Really, Dorothy? Now, a little groggy, I would doze a bit and wake up in a startle—with just moments to dress and drive to the appointed restaurant.

If I were to meet you for dinner at a restaurant, you could be sure of my demure eating disposition. Perhaps a small salad, just a few bites of the high-cholesterol spaghetti carbonara (with leftovers packed in a doggie bag to take home). I would not order dessert but would reluctantly agree to have a taste of yours, followed by a decaf cup of coffee. Agitated by the length of the meal, as my mind was anxiously awaiting the grand buffet awaiting me at home, I would thank you for a wonderful time, grab my doggie bags, and flee back to my own house of ill repute.

Upon entering my house, I would put away the rest of the non-perishable groceries still in the bags from earlier that afternoon and begin designing my binge for the evening. I would check the television lineup, prop up the pillows on my bed, and lay down a sheet on top of my quilt to ensure no crumbs in my bed later—the mark of a seasoned binger. My newest fashion magazines would grace the left side of the bed, although I could fit into nothing that was being advertised, as I prepared for a sugar buffet that would rival the decadent dessert stations at the Four Seasons Hotel. Right-size spoon? Check. Napkins? Check. Milk to go with my cookies (again)? Check. Extra butter theater-style popcorn popping in the microwave? Check. Like a dress rehearsal for a high-society wedding, I had the system set. Once I got into bed to eat, read, and watch TV, I didn't want to have to get up again for anything . . . and I didn't.

Exhausted as I write this, I can now look back and see how draining this whole hamster wheel was. I would eat until I was numb and then sleep poorly (at best) through the night, snoring and with sleep apnea induced by an ever-increasing body size. I would awaken to a mass of destruction—wrappers and spoons and glasses and trays, magazines open, and the TV still on. What had just happened? I don't know if you've ever been burglarized, but a feeling of incredulousness comes over you when you see your whole place vandalized.

Yeah, that's what it's like the morning after—except I was vandalizing me.

Because I can accept that I have addictive behavior concerning food, I am able to seek the right solution for me. I clearly need a highly structured system regarding my food, and I need to be accountable to others each and every day to keep myself honest. While I always viewed myself as an honest person, when it came to food, the only way I could keep my word to myself was to work with others who were experiencing the same kind of food obsession issues I was experiencing.

When I grocery shop today, I sometimes call one of my accountability food friends to alert them—and tell myself—that I'm going into the store to pick up yogurt, oatmeal, four apples, and some chicken. Then I call again when I'm done. I take other actions that support my healthy lifestyle. For example, I now know that if I see too much food porn on television commercials at night, I switch the channel. I do not watch those images and let them get into my brain to create havoc while I sleep. Also, nowadays, if it's 10:00 PM and I'm not attending a special event, I put myself to bed. Imagine that! My mom really did take care of me growing up. She put all the responsible pieces in place for my healthy living, but I just couldn't manage to carry through with them as an adult because I had this addictive behavior bantering about inside.

I used to feel that my addictive behavior would prevent me from future success in business and in life, which is why I refused to believe I had a sugar addiction. Who knew that by finally coming to terms with it, I would implement healthy practices? I now endeavor to take care of myself *because of* the addiction, which has enhanced all areas of my life—including regaining my sporty, athletic, right-size body, of which I am most proud. *Boom!*

Dumpster-Diver Dan

Again, without my even realizing it, one of my hoarding clients came to my rescue. While he had hired me to work with him on his hoarding addiction, by helping him I had another glimpse of how my own addictive behavior was so similar to that of a hoarder.

Dan had it all in his younger life: an executive job, an expensive car, and extreme wealth. Yet, after his father's death, Dan shunned high society, capitalism, and the pretentious lifestyle in which he was raised. He decided to make an extreme "about face" and give it all up. Knowing his history, I would never have expected to share a moment in Dan's life that included Dumpster diving. Waiting for the Cinderella chime at midnight, and only done in the dark of night after most others had gone to sleep, Dan agreed to show me his routine.

From his past life with computers and calculators until now calculating the dive, Dan shared his techniques with me. Wearing miners' headlamps to illuminate the darkness, our hands were free to look for the very special finds at the bottom of the green Dumpster. We scavenged together with city noises screeching in the distance. Dan rescued everything from almost empty bags of cat litter for his cats to already read newspapers from yesterday to slightly broken furniture and electronics, which he was sure he could repair and resell for good money. All of his finds went into his already cramped house, where there was nowhere to sit or sleep. Dan's Dumpster diving gave him a feeling of independence. With little money and no job, he didn't want to depend on family to make it through life. Dan felt a sense of pride when he was able to feed himself with partially bruised fruit and hardened bread from the local deli, which was thrown out at closing time. He knew he was being a good citizen by recycling tattered old clothes and shoes and wearing them rather than sending them off to the local dump station. Dan even felt a sense of heroism when he was able to find computers and other electronics destined for the landfill. He truly felt he was doing a service.

I was able to praise Dan for his conscientiousness about keeping Planet Earth safe, rather than criticize his behavior, as most of his family and neighbors did. I provided the recognition that he was seeking and then began to teach him other recycling techniques that would not hinder his health or his neighbors' homes. His addictive behavior needed attention and intervention. To replace his addiction, Dan later began volunteering at local charity shops and recycling centers, and was able to clean up his home enough to avoid further expensive city fines.

In the midst of this experience, it occurred to me that, like Dan, I also used to go out late at night in search of warm doughnuts or cold ice cream. Just as Dan brought stuff home that no longer fit into his already cramped living quarters, I was buying food to put into an already full body. Though I had just helped another client with his addictive behavior, the similarities to my own addictive eating frightened me.

Current Research on Addiction

I read so many books on cravings and addiction before I found the 12-step program that worked for me, I'm surprised I didn't figure out the answer sooner. Of course, the more I studied, the more shows I did on *Hoarders*, and the more I listened when others spoke of their addictive tendencies, I was able to draw a correlation in my brain to my own addictive behavior. I threw together a simple chart to prove to myself that I was indeed like every other addict out there, and my obsession was food—primarily sugar.

Is Food Addiction Different from Other Addictions?

Food Addiction	Alcoholism	Shopaholism	Hoarding
Just one more cookie	Just one more drink	Just one more purchase	Just one more yard sale
I'll start my diet on Monday—really.	This is my last night; I'm not doing this again.	I won't buy any more after the holidays are over.	Once I fill that back bedroom, it's over; I won't bring in any more.

I must be clear about one thing: I do not represent any particular 12-step group whatsoever. When I speak about these amazing groups, it's only from my perspective, and I cannot be considered —nor claim to be—a spokesperson of any one group. In fact, it is against the traditions of the 12-step world to have spokespeople. Please know that I am just one among many, nobody special, just a gal with her own story to tell, which is why I rely on experts such as Dr. Harold C. Urschel III, founder of the Urschel Recovery Science Institute and author of *Healing the Addicted Brain*. Dr. Urschel writes,

> While we can't say exactly why you become addicted, we do know that there are certain risk factors making one person more susceptible to addiction than another. They include:
>
> - Genetics
> - Emotional state (high levels of stress, anxiety, or emotional pain)
> - Psychological factors (suffering from depression or low self-esteem)
> - Social and cultural factors (having friends or a close partner who displays an activity excessively)
> - Family history (the risk of addiction is higher for people who had a parent or parents who were addicts)

Maia Szalavitz is a health writer at Time.com who interviewed Dr. Gabor Maté. Dr. Maté is highly regarded worldwide for his work in treating people with the worst addictions, most notably at Vancouver's controversial Insite facility, which provides users with clean needles, medical support, and a safe space to inject drugs. Szalavitz asked Dr. Maté how he defines addiction. He replied,

> Any behavior that is associated with craving and temporary relief, and with long-term negative consequences, that a person is not able to give up. Note that I said nothing about substances—it's any behavior that has temporary relief and negative consequences and loss of control. When you look at a process or behavior—sex, gambling, shopping, work, or substances—they engage the same brain circuitry, the same reward system, the same psychological dynamic, and the same spiritual emptiness. People go from one to the other. The issue for me is not whether you're using something or not; it's are you craving, are you needing it for relief, and does it have negative consequences?

How Food Addiction Ties Back to Food and Gaining Weight

When I was heavy into sugar and processed foods, this list of words was always floating through my mind. Can you check off five or more words or phrases that ring true for you from this list? If so, you may want to check your own level of food addiction.

- ✓ Bingeing
- ✓ Buying diet books by the dozen
- ✓ Clothes (especially pants) don't fit
- ✓ Famished
- ✓ Feeling drugged
- ✓ Feeling lazy

✓ Fits of anger

✓ Gorging

✓ Grazing all day and all night

✓ Highly processed foods

✓ Isolation

✓ Night eating

✓ Numbing out

✓ Obsessed with counting calories

✓ One is not enough

✓ Ordering another piece of workout equipment and not using it

✓ Purging

✓ Second helpings

✓ Spending too much money on junk food

✓ Starving

✓ Stashing sugar items

✓ Stomachaches from eating too much

✓ Stopping at drive-throughs a little too often

✓ Sugar-free snacks

✓ Trouble breathing

✓ Twenty-four-hour stores

✓ Way too full

Together with his son, Pax, Chris Prentiss founded Passages Addiction Cure Center in Malibu and wrote *The Alcoholism and Addiction Cure*, which is a holistic approach to recovery. Chris suggests that if you feel depressed for an hour, you've produced approximately 18 billion new cells that have more receptors calling out for more depressed-type peptides. This creates a need for more gloomy thoughts, and you become addicted to gloominess—and therein lies the dependency. In fact, Chris writes that "you'll actually become addicted to that state of being because your body is demanding more of what it is receiving. Addiction, any addiction, is a craving for an emotion. Whether you are addicted to food, sex, shoplifting, or any other compulsive activity, you're engaging in that activity to stimulate a chemical secretion that produces an effect in your brain that brings about the desired sensation, and you're addicted to that sensation."

When I applied Chris's theory to my own food addiction, it made a lot of sense. Though to everyone on the outside it looked like I was punishing myself with food, I was actually seeking what I thought to be an amazing sensation of love and fulfillment. Indeed, I was craving those emotions. Not only was I craving those emotions, but I also began obsessing about food at its very nature. I wondered if I were dreaming, in that everything I saw or heard had something to do with food. Was it some bizarre joke that in just a couple of weeks' time, I heard the following food phrases in everyday conversation?

- If we can get that for free, that's icing on the cake!
- Well, if they include it in the deal, that's just gravy on top!
- Thank you, you really saved my bacon!
- It's like having my cake and eating it, too!
- In order to make it work, we'll need to fudge it a little.
- I just feel like the world is my oyster!
- Are you just trying to butter me up again?
- It's a big project—let's just break it up into bite-size pieces.
- I've just got too much on my plate right now.
- I'm not sure; I'll need to chew on the idea for a bit.
- I can't lose my job—it's my bread and butter.

Before You Begin . . .

Okay, you've heard my story and you know I have a food addiction. To determine if you're at a place in your life where you're ready to address your weight issues, ask yourself the following questions:

1. Are you in the right frame of mind for losing weight?
2. Have you done well with changing your intake of food in the past?
3. Do you like structure?
4. Do you want help from others, or do you succeed best on your own?
5. Are you prepared to make some short-term sacrifices for the long-term goal?
6. What will life be like next year if you don't change your ways?
7. What will life be like in five years if you don't change your ways?
8. What's one thing that is not working for your body (wheezing going up stairs, acid reflux, etc.)?
9. Fast-forward to five years from now. What will that health condition look like?
10. Do you feel you are worth it?

Organizing Tips for Conquering Food Addiction

If you are serious about wanting to lose weight, and you feel like you've tried it all before, here are some tips from the experts and me to help you start your journey. Pick one—any one—and just be open-minded. You never know when your miracle is about to happen. Simply taking action with any of these ten ideas will help shift your energy and put you in the position to stop stuffing your face and start living a healthy life.

TIP 1: *Make a List of Activities You Have Wanted to Do—If Only*

If only I lost weight, I would go dancing more often. If only I lost twenty-five pounds, I would hike on the weekends. If only . . . Stop that! Pick something from your list and do it anyway! Overweight or not, just take action. You'll see that by living life and not putting it off, you just may be inspired to lose the weight. Sitting at home wishing you could dance or hike will get you, um, let's see. . . . Oh! That's right—more of sitting at home. At least by taking a modified hike or dancing, you are experiencing life and increasing your chances to catch the motivation to do something about your weight.

TIP 2: *Discover Your "Bewitching" Hour*

You know, the time you are most likely to go in search of forbidden foods. My times used to be 2:00 PM, 4:00 PM, and 9:00 PM. Developing a clear sense of when you might encounter difficulty can save you from yourself. Once you know your danger times, keep a mental list of alternative activities to redirect you:

Pull out a sketch pad.
Call a friend.
Go get the mail.
Take a hot bath.
Organize your tool bench.
Brush your teeth.
Read one article from a magazine.

TIP 3: *Watch the Documentary* Forks over Knives

This 2011 documentary was directed by independent U.S. film-maker Lee Fulkerson. Through an examination of the careers of

American physician Caldwell Esselstyn and professor of nutritional biochemistry T. Colin Campbell, the film advocates a whole-foods, plant-based (vegan) diet as a means of combating a number of diseases. It suggests that "most, if not all, of the degenerative diseases that afflict us can be controlled, or even reversed, by rejecting our present menu of animal-based and processed foods." The film also provides an overview of the twenty-year China-Cornell-Oxford Project that led to Professor Campbell's findings, outlined in his book *The China Study* (2005), in which he suggests that coronary disease, diabetes, obesity, and cancer can be linked to the Western diet of processed and animal-based foods, including all dairy products.

TIP 4:
Watch the Internet Series The Skinny on Obesity

This series is available at http://www.uctv.tv/skinny-on-obesity/. Robert H. Lustig, MD, and University of California San Francisco professor of pediatrics in the division of endocrinology, explores the damage caused by sugary foods. He argues that fructose (too much) and fiber (not enough) appear to be cornerstones of the obesity epidemic through their effects on insulin. He also has a lecture on sugar that is available at http://www.youtube.com/watch?v=dBnniua6-oM.

TIP 5:
Put Yourself First

What? Yep. I know that most days in my past, I put others' needs first, and by the time I made it home at night, I wanted to be rewarded for it—in food currency. The reward developed into sabotage and later into suffering. What's important to you today? What is something you would like to do that celebrates just you?

TIP 6:
Renegotiate Old Food Agreements with Friends

What do I mean? I used to have certain food rituals saved for certain friends and family members in my life. We had that food item or special drink every time we got together. With my mom, I always had coffee hour with whipped cream and other goodies. It was natural, like clockwork; 4:00 PM came around, and we both knew what to do. Now it's a game of Scrabble instead, and so much more fun.

TIP 7:
Read Lysa TerKeurst

I read a book a few years ago by Lysa TerKeurst, who is the author of fourteen books and encourages nearly half a million women worldwide through a daily online devotional. One of her books, *Made to Crave*, is about satisfying your deepest desire with God, not food. Though I wasn't in the right place to hear anything God-related at the time, I was compelled to read her book, and one particular concept of Lysa's stuck with me. She writes that there is usually a honeymoon phase at the beginning of most eating plans, and something happens—suddenly you're invited to a party. It's a special evening and you justify the pie à la mode by saying you can start again tomorrow, this weekend, or Monday. She explains that it is so tempting to give in and pretend it doesn't matter. In fact, Lysa leads her readers through a new understanding that it does matter, that "We Were Made for More Than This. More than failure, more than this cycle, more than being ruled by taste buds. We were made for victory." I used that mantra for the entire year after reading it, and I really came to believe that I was made for more than just another bag of overprocessed cookies. My cravings began to shift. Perhaps yours will, too.

TIP 8:
Be Compassionate with Yourself and Others

According to Dr. Harold Urschel, as a general rule, it takes at least six to ten months of sobriety or abstinence before significant brain repair is achieved. The disease of addiction has no quick fixes, which is why addicts deserve sympathy and support, even when they lapse.

TIP 9:
Learn About Cravings

Dr. Mike Dow is the cohost of VH1's *Couples Therapy*, host of TLC's *My 600-Pound Life* special, host of TLC's *Freaky Eaters*, and author of *Diet Rehab*. He is also the clinical director of therapeutic and behavioral services at the Body Well integrative medical center in Los Angeles. Dr. Dow authored the book *Diet Rehab: 28 Days to Stop Craving the Foods that Make You Fat*. He says that cravings can be your worst enemy when you're trying to lose weight. And what a lot of people don't know is that certain foods can fuel cravings even more, making it harder to resist them. Luckily, Dr. Dow has a twenty-eight-day plan to stop you from craving the foods that make you gain weight. His plan uses techniques that help retrain your brain to desire foods that fill you up and keep you healthy rather than empty foods that won't satiate your hunger. For example, he says, "Salt is one of the worst craving offenders. It plays tricks on your taste buds, raises blood pressure, and generally triggers cravings for unhealthy, sodium-rich foods. Instead of using salt as a seasoning, try any of these other kinds of seasonings as a healthier alternative: black pepper, basil, cilantro, curry, ginger, oregano, paprika, rosemary, sage, or turmeric."

TIP 10:
Use E-Learning Tools

Dr. Urschel says that addicts must learn to handle cravings, attend 12-step meetings regularly, and otherwise revamp their thinking, behavior, and lifestyle. To get comprehensive and innovative e-learning tools that provide in-depth addiction education and support, visit www.EnterHealth.com/Healing theAddictedBrain.

Twelve-Step Programs

By the time I was forty, I had never been to a 12-step meeting, nor had I ever been exposed to the concept of 12-step work. Even so, I found my personal answers to my weight problems in a 12-step program. That particular program, and all others, were an outgrowth from the original program of Alcoholics Anonymous. A 2011 article in the *Scientific American Mind*, written by Hal Arkowitz and Scott O. Lilienfeld, reported that Alcoholics Anonymous counted 2 million members who participated in some 115,000 groups worldwide, about half of them in the United States. The duo researched how well the 12-step program worked.

Anthropologist William Madsen, then at the University of California, Santa Barbara, claimed in a 1974 book that it has a "nearly miraculous" success rate, whereas others are far more skeptical. After reviewing the literature, we found that AA may help some people overcome alcoholism, especially if they also get some professional assistance, but the evidence is far from overwhelming, in part because of the nature of the program.

In AA, members meet in groups to help one another achieve and maintain abstinence from alcohol. The meetings, which are free and open to anyone serious about stopping drinking, may include reading from the Big Book, sharing stories, celebrating members' sobriety, as well as discussing the 12 steps and themes related to problem drinking. Participants are encouraged to "work" the 12-step program, fully integrating each step into their lives before proceeding to the next. AA targets more than problem drinking; members are supposed to correct all defects of character and adopt a new way of life.

In a 2012 *Oprah* magazine article about how age brings perspective, seventy-eight-year-old Shirley MacLaine was asked to give some advice to her twenty-five-year-old self. She wrote, "Dear Shirley, Regardless of how outrageous it may seem, ask for guidance from your higher self and follow it. Also, don't eat so much sugar."

Dorothy the Organizer's Six-Week Body Declutter Plan

Whether you're a packrat or a calorie counter, a neat freak or a binge eater, to be successful on the scale, you must first master the clutter within you and around you. My Six-Week Body Declutter Plan gives you the tools to declutter your way to your right size by transforming and adopting new ways of thinking, feeling, and acting by facing the stuff in your life. Whether it's an obsession with food or issues with self-esteem, whether you're struggling with your finances or too much clutter, whether you're in need of a community or need to commune with God, this plan can get you started.

Week 1: Assess and Prepare

Week 2: Pick Your Tools

Week 3: Join a Group

Week 4: Parent Yourself

Week 5: Fill in the Blanks

Week 6: Connect to Your Universal Life Force

Week 1: Assess and Prepare

✓ Pull out a notebook. Write down your height, age, weight, and the date.

✓ Look around your house, apartment, or room for signs: clutter, unopened mail, clothing not hung on hangers, dead plants, unwashed dishes, rings in the tub and toilet, kitty litter unchanged, laundry piling up—make an assessment. Take notes. Later, as a diversion from eating, you will begin to address these neglected areas.

✓ Look at yourself in the mirror. Start at the top of your body and work your way down. Do you need a haircut, a pair of glasses, dental work? When is the last time you had a mammogram? Are your nails trimmed? Do your undies fit properly? Take a look at you and the condition you're in. What needs attention? Make your notes and hold on to them; you'll need them to remind you to take care of you.

✓ Check the kitchen cabinets and fridge for contraband (the foods and high-sugar drinks that you feel you shouldn't be eating and drinking). If you want to make a positive shift today, you've got to give yourself a fighting chance. Remove the temptation.

✓ Put the bathroom scale away. Weighing yourself daily can set you up for daily disappointments. Make a decision to weigh yourself once a week—preferably once a month. You'll leave the obsession of the scale behind and focus on more important activities. If you feel a scale is essential, invest in a food scale instead.

Week 2: Parent Yourself

✓ You may or may not have children. You may or may not
    have had consistent parenting as a child. However, if you are
    carrying too much weight or are obsessed with food thoughts
    regularly, it is time to step in and parent yourself. This means
    listening to an inner voice, a voice that knows better, in terms
    of nurturing yourself. Your adult self may need to consider
    telling your young self to get to bed earlier, not to eat so
    much sugar, and to do your homework.

✓ Make your food quantities consistent. For example, many
    of us are accustomed to meat portion sizes of 8–10 ounces
    when the recommended portion is just 2–4 ounces of cooked
    meat, poultry, or fish (minus the bones, skin, and fat). When
    you eat an 8-ounce portion, your tummy expects the same
    amount at its next meal. Your brain becomes trained to want
    it, and your body is trained to consume it. If you happen to
    skip a meal to make up for overeating, your brain and body
    scream (i.e., crave) even louder and stronger, and your next
    meal becomes a round-the-world international food fest.
    Consistency is key here. Try to design the same portions or
    measurements for most of your meals.

Week 3: Join a Group

✓ Stop having conversations with yourself and start talking
    with others. Having conversations with other like-minded
    people will put you in a place of belonging and being
    understood. You can be part of my FaceYourStuff Club, join
    Weight Watchers, or attend any number of 12-step programs.
    For a list of 12-step groups to consider, visit the Resources
    section at the back of the book.

Week 4: Pick Your Tools

✓ Plan your food and write it down in your notebook. Decide in advance what you plan to eat each day. Similar to shopping, if you create a list before you go, you are likely to stick to the list and not overspend or buy items you do not need. The same is true for your food consumption. If you spell out what you plan to eat for the day in advance, the more likely you are to stick to it.

✓ Know your enemies. Get clear now on the foods that call you and the places that lure you in. For example, anything I can pop into my mouth quickly (and in multiples) is a no-no for me. Nuts, mini-chocolates, grapes, popcorn—all way too easy and way too dangerous for me.

Week 5: Fill in the Blanks

✓ Educate yourself with information that supports your new healthy lifestyle.

✓ Manage boredom and the urge to eat by making a list of things to do, other than eat. Remember that assessment you did back in Week 1? Now's the time to steer clear of the food and do something else. You can also create a list of fun things to do as well!

✓ Rather than nibbling, end your evening by reading an inspirational message or mantra.

Week 6: Connect to Your Universal Life Force

✓ Begin a prayer regimen that fits into your concept of a Universal Life Force even if you don't "believe." Ask your ULF to help you eat healthy today, make sensible decisions, and take responsible actions.

✓ Once a day, make a list of ten things for which you are grateful. Our universal laws say that when we focus on the gratitude we feel for what we do have rather than focusing on what we don't have, we experience happier moments, have less stress, and attract more goodness into our lives.

✓ Check out Ann Voskamp's *New York Times* bestselling book, *One Thousand Gifts: A Dare to Live Fully Right Where You Are*. There's a great daily devotional and study guide available, too.

Organizing Tips for Healthy Eating and Exercise

Over the last decade, my business partner Debby Bitticks, a nationally recognized intergenerational expert, made a great impact in my life toward reexamining what healthy living looked like for me. Because of this, Debby was the first contributor whom I turned to when writing this book. Debby breaks down healthy eating for all of us. Here are her easy tips for helping you stay organized and feeling good.

Easy Tips for Organizing Meals (at Home, at Work, in Restaurants, at Social Events, and When Traveling)

At Home

- Keep fresh vegetables and fruits available and where they are in easy view.
- Cook several days' worth of a protein (like white meat chicken or fish) and cut it up in chunks so that you can instantly throw it into a salad or soup and have a healthy snack or meal.
- Keep very few items in the house that contain sugar.

- Maintain a gluten-free shelf or a lactose-free shelf, depending on your personal needs.
- Prepare little Ziplock bags with measured snacks ready to eat.

At Work

Carry a thermal bag (looks like a purse) and always have fruit, vegetables, and a protein with you. Remember to bring healthy snacks. Because the bag keeps things cold, if you go out for lunch, your food stays fresh and comes home with you at the end of the day.

In Restaurants

When I know in advance that I am going to a restaurant, I go online and study the menu. I think ahead about what I will order. If I have a question, I call the restaurant and tell them I'm coming for lunch or dinner and ask for their help in what I can order due to my food allergies. I almost always find them to be helpful. With no advance notice when I'm in a restaurant, I ask and thank the server for helping me select a meal that I can eat. Again, I almost always find them eager to be helpful. Just in case, I always carry a protein bar and healthy snack in my purse and briefcase.

At Social Events

I have told most of my friends, family, and colleagues that I have food allergies and everyone is supportive and helpful. By thinking ahead and being organized, I usually don't need to inconvenience anyone. Example: The children of one of our friends invited my husband and me to a rather formal fiftieth wedding anniversary party for our friends. Rather than contacting them, I called the catering department at the country club and explained that I was going to attend the event. I asked the catering director to speak to the kitchen staff about what was being served and explained my health issues. We worked out a plan where my salmon would be served to me without the gluten sauce (just with lemon) and they would provide steamed vegetables and fruit. With no extra charge to the host, and no disruption whatsoever at the dinner, I simply told the server at my table that I was Debby and the kitchen had a special meal for me. I brought my own gluten-free cookies for dessert and enjoyed a wonderful anniversary celebration. My husband also usually carries snacks in his jacket for me.

When Traveling

When traveling by car I keep a large cold food container in the car filled with my healthy foods and drinks. If I stop at a restaurant and don't need the food, it remains cold and fresh. However, knowing that I have it with me always helps to keep me calm, secure, and prepared.

When flying, I carry my purse-looking thermal food bag. Knowing that I have healthy foods and snacks keeps me from being hungry or getting into a situation where eating the wrong foods could make me feel ill and affect my trip. Also, I carry a note from my doctor that states that I need to have special food with me for health reasons. That way my food bag is not considered luggage; I can still carry my purse and carry-on suitcase.

I also always call ahead to the hotel and ask to have a small refrigerator in my room. I carry protein bars, an avocado, snacks, and a banana in my luggage.

When I'm staying with family, I send an e-mail list ahead of time so they know what I need. I also find out what types of markets and restaurants are located near their home. I can easily have my list ready and go to the store and get what I need. Being organized in advance creates a peaceful feeling that helps me enjoy my loved ones without food issues interfering.

How Many Gym Memberships
Does It Take to Make You Skinny?

Since I'm kind of "telling on myself" in this book so far, I guess I'll uncover the equally embarrassing secret about all the money I spent on gym memberships. You may know the internal thought process. For me it was, *Hmm, it's the end of July and I never got into my bikini as I'd planned. I know—I'll join a gym! It's on my way to work, I'll stop in every morning, and* boom! *I'll finally get this extra weight off my body.* Ever had a conversation like this with yourself? Let me share more of mine.

First week—*Super! The gym workout is exhausting but I'm doing it.*

Second week—*My gym workout is still exhausting, and honestly, it's not so convenient doing it before I go to work. I have to bring all of my clothes and shower there (and the gym bag that I purchased to support this idea isn't quite the right one).* I manage going only four days a week now.

Third week—*Wow, I'm still eating like crazy at work due to stress, and going to the gym doesn't seem to be helping the same way it did when I was a gymnast. Frankly, the parking at the gym in the morning is a disaster. I can never get a spot, and I'm kind of late getting up out of bed (Translation: I don't want to go), and, well, all of that makes me late for work.*

If those excuses weren't enough, I'd design another strategy instead: *Let's see, I know. There is another gym that is much closer to home and is far less expensive. I don't think I can get out of my contract at the first gym, but I really need to get into shape. I know it sounds stupid, but I could negotiate a shorter-term contract with this new gym and could make it all work.*

Yep, my insanity had its way with me. I just wanted to lose the weight, and I didn't have the full answer to my lifelong struggle with food yet. Have you ever done anything as ridiculous as this? Looking back, I would be too embarrassed to add up all the money spent on gym memberships and other contraptions to get the doggone weight off my body.

For some of you, exercise may be the answer, however. If it is, Kipling Solid, who holds a degree in corporate fitness, may be able to help. She currently owns Solid Bodies, a personal training and Pilates studio, and has combined experience of twenty-plus years in the fitness industry. When it comes to health and fitness, Kipling has a few things to share with us:

Being a teacher of exercise, I've learned to embody movement. I teach clients autonomy in their own bodies. My goal is to allow them to embody movement and apply it wherever they go in their journey. Everyone already comes equipped with mind, body, and spirit. Self-awareness, managing emotions, motivation, and empathy are all areas I've been working on for a lifetime. As a trainer I can pass the baton, step back, and watch a beautiful transformation in you!

My number-one requirement when a client comes to me: Have fun! Second on my list: Don't get hurt! Whether it is your trainer or you making the decision to exercise, know your own limits. More important, use your voice and speak up. No one can do that for you. Trainers are your guide. We come alongside you to propel you into a place you weren't aware existed. Your limits are only your own. Below are a few suggestions in terms of getting your body moving again—the key is to get it moving.

Cardio: Five Times per Week

- Start with any activity you can maintain for fifteen minutes, eventually working up to forty-five minutes.
- Combine walking and cycling.
- Stair climbing or elliptical reflects variation of movement.
- I don't recommend running unless you feel compelled to start or continue.

- The goal is longevity—do things that don't antagonize injuries but make you stronger.

Strength Training: Three Times per Week

- Use weights that you can manage.
- Use all muscle groups: chest, back, arms, legs.
- It is not necessary to do more than eight repetitions of anything, as it increases risk for injury.
- Proper form always comes before adding resistance.
- Find a reliable source who can advise you. A professional opinion is definitely worth the cost of preventing injury.

Core

Everyone is talking about strengthening their core. Working the core is part of conditioning the whole body. I've come across a great mind-bending definition by my mentor in Pilates: "'Core' is a condition, not a location." The second powerhouse or group of muscles that help stabilize and align the abs are located in the shoulder girdle. This group comprises the rear deltoids, external rotators, rhomboids, triceps, latissmus dorsi, and serratus. The serratus is only as strong as the diaphragm's ability to move freely in the belly. You want strong abs? Start practicing breathing through your primary breathing muscle. Your diaphragm is the only way to expand your breath into oxygenating the body. Practice your breath daily:

- Lie on your back.
- Place hands on belly.
- Inhale and exhale through the nose.
- Feel belly rise and lower.
- You will feel less dizzy over time as you become better at breathing.

Pilates

Core and breathing takes us right into Pilates, an exercise program created by Joseph Pilates. What is Pilates? The basic answer is whole-body exercise. Pilates applies to both powerhouses mentioned earlier: strengthening the core and practiced breathing. The apparatus or equipment used in Pilates works with springs under tension, which causes more or less effort depending on the amount of springs loaded.

The springs work by creating effort against the muscles that actively push back against the springs. The stronger you become in Pilates, the fewer springs you use. Anyone can participate in Pilates. Don't let anybody say otherwise. Just be sure to speak up if anything hurts you. The last thing you want is to walk away from Pilates saying that your neck hurts. A good teacher will make accommodations if something hurts. Finally, remember that Pilates can be practiced apart from using equipment at studios or gyms. Many books and DVDs do not involve studio equipment but still apply the Pilates methods.

Accountability

Accountability is your responsibility to show up for your own health. I will show up for you in terms of training, but will *you* be there for you? In my opinion, your good health is not an option. Finally, remember that humor is key to longevity in life. In my book, there is no frowning in exercise or Pilates! My kids run downstairs and peek into my studio, wondering what could be so hilarious, and I say, "It's just another day at the office." Keep your attitude upbeat and laugh often. How's that for a fitness routine?

Dorothy's Experts Weigh
In on the Matter

Over the years, I have to admit, I've tried so many diets, technologies, methods, practices, systems, and weight-loss programs—from hypnosis to a "Suck Your Fat Off with a Vacuum" product—and *they all worked*! But because I was an unidentified food addict, all of these trials and successes did not last. However, one of these approaches may work for you, and I want to be sure you have the opportunity to try them, too. I want to thank each and every expert for creating their system for me to try. Their work is worthy, and today I am using one or more tools from their creations in my daily life. Since not all of you come from the perspective of food addiction, you may want to try some other solutions with one of my former weight-loss gurus. Here's a bit of information to whet your brain appetite about each of the approaches I tried.

You on a Diet: The Owner's Manual
for Waist Management

I love this book by Dr. Roizen and Dr. Oz! It works! Here's why I read it cover to cover. The authors taught me that it was my waist circumference and not my overall weight that is the most important indicator of mortality related to being overweight. They taught me that I needed to switch from focusing on the pounds on a scale to the inches on my tape measure. Because of its proximity to your organs, state Drs. Oz and Roizen, your belly fat is the most dangerous fat you carry. This book starts you off with a "Fat Facts Test" accompanied by oodles of hysterically funny and very informative illustrations.

Several other factors in this book were also very helpful, such as the information that "the battle over eating isn't between your willpower and the Belgian waffles; it's between your brain chemicals," and the authors' explanation for how to figure out how stressed I was: "Take a look at how much belly fat you have. The larger your waist, the higher your stress." If you relate to any of these powerful thoughts, this book is for you.

The Body You Deserve: Weight-Loss Strategies for a Vital Lifestyle

In this particular set of CDs and workbooks by Anthony Robbins, I learned about interrupting my old patterns and how to transform my vocabulary. Tony suggests avoiding the "Language of Failure" in favor of using the "Language of Success." Using language like "I'm starving, I'm famished, I'm dying for a burger" doesn't lead to the kind of behavior you want. He feels that with the Language of Success, you can talk about your pride, dignity, strength, endurance, commitment, and passion. Additionally, Tony gives readers and listeners Morning Power Questions, Evening Power Questions, and Problem-Solving Questions. For me, these questions alone were the most effective part of his system, and I still use them today. Perhaps this system can inspire you, too.

The Ultimate Weight-Loss Solution: The Seven Keys to Weight-Loss Freedom

Not only have I met Dr. Phil and been on his show, I take his advice. In this book, Dr. Phil delivers seven keys to weight-loss freedom, and I especially related to Key No. 3: Create a No-Fail Environment. Dr. Phil believes that it is necessary for you to shape, design, and manage your environment so that it is virtually impossible for you to fail at weight control. He feels that concentrating on the personal landscape of your life, which includes everything from your home to your office, must be cleaned up in order for you to lose weight. He suggests burning all "external bridges" that invite needless snacking, overeating, and bingeing. Getting rid of clothes from your plus-size life was my take-away from this book. Never again would I allow myself to hold on to my "fat clothes" just in case. Perhaps Dr. Phil's direct approach could work for you.

The 4-Hour Body: An Uncommon Guide to Rapid Fat-Loss, Incredible Sex, and Becoming Superhuman

No, seriously, if you want radical, uncommon, superhuman results, then you might consider this book by Timothy Ferriss. Tim is irreverent, super curious, clever, funny, and a doer. Tim quotes comedian Ed Bluestone early in his book: "I have a great diet. You're allowed to eat anything you want, but you must eat it with naked fat people." Despite his humorous approach, Tim also suggests that you must find a weight-loss method that works for you, even if it's less effective and less efficient than you would like. He says that the decent method you follow is better than the perfect method you quit. What resonated most for me with Tim's book is his excellent research, both in his own experimentation and in academic study. He comes to the table with common mistakes and misunderstandings and how to live a longer and better life. Tim's book is worth the read—if you dare.

I've got to tell you, each of these books worked for me; it's just that in the past, when I tried these various methods, I was usually reading the book or trying the system because I had some upcoming event. By an upcoming event, I mean a hometown class reunion, an upcoming vacation that required looking good in a bathing suit, or entering a Miss Petite America beauty pageant (no, I am not joking; I entered this pageant in my twenties).

Always seeking to try again, I picked up the book *Thin Within: How to Eat and Live Like a Thin Person* by Judy Wardell a couple of months prior to the pageant. Excellent book! I had huge success. Her book had food-tracking logs, success tools, and an "Observations and Corrections" chart. I noted whether I ate when I was hungry, whether I ate in a calm environment, whether I was sitting or standing, and I confirmed that I ate and drank only the things my body loved. Per the book's instructions, I ate slowly, and I stopped before my body was full.

Pageant day arrived, and I was thirty pounds thinner. One interview, one bathing suit competition, and one ball-gown face-off later, I landed in the top five finalists. That tiara was just out of reach for me, but I left the pageant feeling kind of sexy and full of confidence, and what better way to celebrate than by going out for a scrumptious meal followed by elegant desserts? Yep, that's plural. Not even a week later, I had quickly gained back ten of the thirty pounds. In another month I was in worse shape than before I had started my weight-loss journey. The insanity wouldn't leave me alone, though. If I'd blown all that hard work, endured all the positive attention about my weight loss, and then suffered the bulging eyes and frowns from others about my weight gain, I figured, *Why bother at all?* My pattern was as predictable as my morning alarm clock. Social event coming soon? Diet. Celebrate! Binge. Retreat. Isolate. New event? Diet, binge . . . well, you get the idea.

After I had my epiphany watching my own *Hoarders*® episode, I decided to lose weight finally, and I joined a program. I realized it was not a quick fix to slim the waistline but a way of *totally* rethinking my life, relationships, and spirituality; I needed to do this to stay alive, happy, and healthy. This time there was no event to go to, no diet to be implemented, nothing to celebrate, and no reason to binge, retreat, or isolate anymore. Here's what happened:

You know how some people can make a decision to quit smoking and then just do it? Others decide to give up caffeine for good and make it happen? I could never understand how they were able to make such a life change. I knew it could never happen to me—but I was wrong. If you feel that way about yourself, I would like to go out on a limb and say that maybe you are wrong, too. A massive life change can happen for you. There is hope for all of us here. That shift, especially about our weight and our bodies, may never come when we want it to, but if we keep even just a glimmer of hope, it will eventually happen for us.

A few years ago, I was nearly 200-plus pounds, and the most amazing guy appeared in my life. We met at a business function, and he asked me out for dinner. In the back of my mind, I asked him, *Can't you see that I'm incredibly overweight? Should I stand up again so that you can see what you're getting here?* Instead, I said yes. Friends told me that he probably asked me out because I was a bright entrepreneur with a bold outlook, a contagious smile, and trusting eyes. I didn't realize it then, but this relationship would become the single most important dating relationship I would ever have.

For the first time in my life, I found myself in a relationship with someone I absolutely trusted. Steve always called when he said he would, held confidences for me and others like a vault, was truthful about his feelings, and was a man of his word. I just didn't know what that was like. My therapist, Sharma, told me that I had to keep dating to work through all of my old hurt and trauma, and one day, I would be done with it all. Steve helped me to "be done with it all," and I cannot thank him enough for it.

Steve and I dated for two years, and during that time, I was able to express myself clearly about what I wanted in the relationship and so was he. Because I could trust him, I didn't need to run home to eat secretly anymore. Slowly, the weight was beginning to come off my body, not because I was dieting or over-exercising or seeing a hypnotist (yes, I went this route, too). It was coming off because I had found a place and a person with whom I could be honest.

Now, honesty can hurt. I wanted a permanent relationship with Steve, and he was "just fine" with the way our relationship was. We couldn't come to an agreement as to the future of our relationship, and for the first time I broke up with a guy without there being any trauma (well, except for my endless sobbing). There was no jail time here, no other women, no misuse of money, no misunderstandings or arguments—it was truly just a parting of the ways. Never before had I had such an experience.

I didn't know how to react. I wasn't angry or catatonic or feeling spiteful. Yes, I was hurting, but I wasn't being driven to eat. I just needed someone to understand me and nurture me. I went to Mom, which I had rarely done before because of my pride. I showed up at her door in a complete blob of tears. I finally let her in far enough to help—a grown-up thing to do. She didn't say much, just put me on the couch and boiled some tea bags to place on my bulging, tear-filled eyes. My sister Pat sat at the end of the couch and rubbed my feet. None of us really said anything. I just cried, and they just nurtured. It's the first time I can ever remember such family love—not that folks weren't willing to give it; I had just finally learned to accept it. Such sweetness. A couple of hours later, Steve called to check on me; nothing was changing, but he is a deeply kind man who went the extra distance to make sure I was okay.

My next stop was a 12-step program. A colleague of mine attended such meetings, and I resolved to go, too. I asked my sister to go with me, and we walked into a brightly lit hospital conference room filled with warm, welcoming, thoughtful people. I listened as others read about the 12 steps.

It was enough to keep me interested. I continued to go back to more meetings because I wanted to surround myself with like-minded, positive, do-something-about-your-situation kind of people. Truly, I was no longer seeking just to eliminate the fat on my body; I wanted answers and a way of life that I could implement for good. I needed to accept that I was addicted to certain foods and learn how to become humble and grateful. I had to relearn how to be on time, be helpful to others, and cultivate a concept about spirituality—something I had never tried to do before in my life.

Though I want to talk endlessly about my 12-step experience, I must keep it short. The basic tenet for all 12-step programs is that its members remain anonymous. I cannot and do not consider myself a spokesperson for any 12-step program, but I can share that this approach worked for me. Over the next year and a half, I worked my program and released more than seventy-five pounds—and have kept it off. We all get our chance at this miracle regarding our struggle. We simply can *never, never* give up. Do not give up, my friends. I've waited nearly fifty years for this experience. If you haven't been able to make it happen, hang in there. It will come. You will be okay.

Current Research on Weight Gain and Weight Loss

From a remarkable one-hour video featured at ABC.net (http://www.abc.net.au/news/2012-07-24/globesity—fats-new-frontier/4151576), I learned the term "globesity." This video reports the following:

> The world is getting very fat, very fast, and now the obesity epidemic has spread from rich countries to poor and developing countries, and it is likely 1 billion people will be obese by 2030. Fat is being called the new tobacco. Body weight is not just about vanity, it is about life and death, with obesity increasing the risk of heart disease, type-2 diabetes, and some forms of cancer. So how and why did the problem of obesity explode in places that, not so long ago, counted malnutrition and even famine as major health concerns? Well, it's about increasing wealth, changing diets, genetic programming, and aggressive marketing by international food companies. In our special examination of arguably the world's number-one health issue, "Globesity: Fat's New Frontier," a foreign correspondent visits the new obesity hotspots—Mexico, Brazil,

China, and India—where hundreds of millions are gripped by weight issues and associated diseases. The most perplexing problem in emerging economies is how they are going to deal with a tidal wave of obesity with relatively scant health resources.

The producers of the video canvassed opinions from notable authorities on diet, nutrition, and fat issues, and met people in these countries who are struggling with the consequences of obesity. It's an eye-opening, sometimes shocking journey. Writer Carrie Gann wrote an online piece for ABC.net in which she asked the question, "Is sugar as dangerous as alcohol and tobacco?" Her investigation shows, "One group of researchers from the University of California, San Francisco, says so. And they are urging a tax on sugary treats and some action by the government to get Americans to cut back on sugar."

Gann further reported that "in an editorial published in the journal *Nature*, the UCSF doctors Robert Lustig, Laura Schmidt, and Claire Brindis said, 'The ballooning rates—and costs—of obesity, diabetes, and other diseases mean it's time for regulators to lump sugar into the same category as booze and cigarettes and put similar restrictions on its sale and availability.' Increased control is necessary, they say, because efforts to keep excessive sugar out of the American diet have failed."

Dr. Margaret Christensen graduated cum laude with degrees in biology and psychology. She received her medical degree from Baylor College of Medicine in Houston, and she received her board certification as a fellow of the American College of Obstetrics and Gynecology. In 2001 she was called by Spirit to close her traditional practice and take a two-year sabbatical for research, transformative growth, and profound personal healing.

By integrating and applying her findings on creating health into her own life, she now helps inspire her clients to do the same. In her new practice, the Christensen Center for Whole Life Health, she combines the latest scientific research together with healing wisdom and teachings from many traditions. When asked the question, "Why can't I lose weight?" Dr. Christensen says,

Managing to lose and maintain a healthy weight is a huge issue for many women. Unfortunately three of the main factors that cause excessive weight gain are never addressed by yo-yo and fad diets. These three factors are *hormonal imbalances*, *inflammation*, and *toxicity*. These three factors in turn are exacerbated by lack of nutrients, unhealthy bacteria in the gut, stress, lack of sleep, and lack of movement.

Most weight-loss schemes create more long-term stress on the body because they are not addressing the underlying disturbances. Thus, you may lose weight initially, but it all comes back, plus more, because you have altered the body composition unfavorably. Scale weight is not an indicator of a woman's body fat or health. Looking thin is not necessarily a sign that you are healthy. What we are interested in is a healthy body composition, that is, increasing lean body mass, which is metabolically active (burns calories), while decreasing total percent of body fat (burns no calories).

Lean body weight is the total mass of everything in your body—bones, muscles, organs, water, and so on, except for fat. Since lean mass weighs more than fat, you may not lose as much weight on the scale; however, you are leaner, more fit, and have a healthier metabolism. Over the long run this will help you achieve your ideal weight, create healthier cells, and improve your overall well-being.

It takes, on average, five to seven years to replace all of the cells in your body—you are literally made out of what you consume (at all levels). How you look and feel five years from now is dependent on what you are putting into your body today. Treating inflammation through a detoxification process helps rid your body of both external and internal toxins that may be interfering with your metabolism and ability to lose weight while at the same time providing the body with the healthy ingredients and necessary nutrients to create healthy new cells.

When we look at what affects our health and weight, our lifestyle is the biggest factor. When we eat more calories than we burn from lack of physical activity and high-fat, high-sugar diets, we experience weight gain, especially if we are under chronic, low-grade stress. Cortisol produced during stress triggers food cravings and fat storage, particularly if elevated at night. Sleep quantity and quality play a huge role in weight maintenance—adequate sleep in the diurnal rhythm humans were evolved with (bed at darkness, up with dawn).

It is critically important to eat protein for breakfast; it will help maintain an even blood glucose level throughout the day, decreasing cravings and total calorie consumption. As a human species we are designed to expend our energy most efficiently with movement throughout the day. So if you don't move the energy that is coming in, then it will get "stuck" on your thighs, stomach, and buttocks. You have to move it, if you want to lose it!

Emotional health also plays a major role in helping us understand and change our unhealthy eating patterns. Most of know what we should do, we just have a hard time implementing it. Using a tool such as Emotional Freedom Technique (EFT), or "tapping," can help change underlying sabotaging behavioral patterns.

3

DO YOU HAVE A CLUTTER PROBLEM?

Unearth Your "Stuff" to Get Your Ideal-Size Body Back

I had three experiences in life that taught me how to manage my clutter (other than my mom showing me how—have I thanked you for *that* one yet, Mom?): (1) At age thirty I traveled around the world for a year with just a backpack. (2) Upon my divorce I had to sell everything I owned, including my three-bedroom house, to pay for the services of a PR firm to help me get my business on the map. (3) I began filming *Hoarders*®.

Now, wait a second. I don't want you to get the wrong idea. I have always been quite organized and have had considerable training in the subject. However, there were significant moments in my life when I had life-changing brain shifts while dealing with stuff and clutter. The first was when I returned from my trip around the world and looked at all of my belongings differently. Having visited home after home in many Eastern Bloc and Third World countries, I no longer wanted to have such excess in my home. While what I had was indeed organized, I simply had too much for my taste. After I unpacked from my journey, it was just a few days before I began the vital review of stuff in the upstairs of my home and started deleting unnecessary items from floor to floor. By the time I had reached the basement, I had enough stuff to set up a second apartment for someone. I sold it all. The clutter doctor—my alter ego—was in, and this was just my first appointment.

My second appointment with this alter ego was right after my divorce. Just months after Bob and I split, I found myself facing the consequences of his behavior. As a woman of financial integrity and refusing to declare bankruptcy due to his unbelievable life choices, I began my climb out of sudden and severe financial debt. Simultaneously, I needed to make a name for myself in the organizing industry or retreat back immediately to my nine-to-five secretarial job at UCLA. Determined and believing that making it was my only answer, I hired a top-tier PR agent. Once I signed an agreement with my PR agent, I knew I had to come up with some big bucks every month to cover his fee and all the expenses that go along with creating a brand. I looked around at all my stuff and began to create a "points value system." Number 5 was the highest value number in my point system.

Dorothy the Organizer's "Points Value System" for Rating Stuff

5 If an item ranked a 5 in terms of importance, it was nonnegotiable and it stayed: my green-stained Depression glass, my photos, my business files and office equipment, my car.

4 Number 4 on the scale represented things that were difficult to replace and items I used every day: most of my clothes, music CDs, some furniture, a favorite set of sheets and towels, jewelry.

3 See no. 1.

2 See no. 1.

1 From there I went straight to items that I considered a 1 on the scale: items I never used—seasonal items, specialized tools, or kitchen gadgets. I got rid of pretty stationery, extra wrapping paper, boxes for shipping something someday, specialized boxes I kept as original packaging for my television, printer, and electric can opener. Gone, gone, gone.

That left me with numbers 2 and 3 on my scale of keep or toss. You know what I found? There really were no items that rated 2 or 3 on my scale. Once I established some criteria questions, I was able to sort and purge like never before. I asked myself,

- Do I love it?
- What's the special story behind it?
- Do I have the space for it?
- Can it be replaced?
- Can I easily borrow it or rent it if I need it again?
- Does it compare to the other items that are ranked in the number 5 position?

I looked at my life. I knew my priority was to start my business, and that meant I needed to sell my house to make it happen. I kept the bigger goal in sight and created the criteria for keeping or letting go of stuff that would not support that goal. What I didn't know then was that I was practicing what I was going to preach. I learned organizing from the bottom up, or as my very famous and brilliant colleague Julie Morgenstern says, "Organizing from the Inside Out," which is also the title of her fabulous book on how to get organized.

You Can't Take It with You

When we come to the end of our lives, we take no material items with us. We take not one precious penny in our cold, dead hands. The only thing we take with us is knowing that we have helped others. If we have given our time and money, we take this peace with us. Looking back at your life, what are you proud of? Those are the things that really matter in the long run—not our stuff.

One of the top reasons for mounds of clutter is indecision, says my very insightful organizing colleague, affectionately known as the Paper Tiger Lady, Barbara Hemphill. Whether it's paper or any other item that requires a decision, I suggest you "TAPP it." I have created a technique called TAPP (Toss, Act, Pile or file, Pass it on) to manage all of your paper decisions. I use this acronym all the time to help my clients learn how to make quick decisions on their own about any item in their home or office. Let's say I can't make a decision about a graduation invitation that's come in the mail. I simply visualize TAPP and run through my choices, as follows:

T (Toss)	I could toss the invitation. I don't like the kid who's graduating, I've never like the kid, and I'm not going to go to the graduation.
A (Act on it)	I do something with the invitation. I actually like the kid; I want to go to the graduation. I RSVP. I buy a card, write a check, and keep it in a file marked "Graduation—June 20."
P (Pile it)	Yeah, I still don't like the kid, but I *love* the graduation announcement. I think I'll keep it in my idea pile (or file) and use

something similar for my daughter's
graduation next year!

P (Pass it on) You know, pass it on to someone else. Get
it out of my space! I don't know the kid, but
my husband and son know him through
the basketball team. I'll give it to them
to handle.

> **Trying to be happy by accumulating possessions
> is like trying to satisfy hunger by taping
> sandwiches all over your body.**
>
> —*George Carlin*

Something else to consider is that our culture is a huge source of
stress. Do you happen to know the average amount of time Americans spend shopping per week? Do you want to venture a guess?
According to recent data from the American Time Use Survey,
nearly six hours! What happened? Stuff happened. Bigger homes,
fewer children. More room for more stuff. And our culture provides
us with countless opportunities and choices to be busier and collect
more stuff than ever before.

We go to trade shows and collect stuff. We go to classes and
seminars and receive paper and binders. We pick up freebies and
promotional items; we go shopping, host kids' activities, travel, open
mounds of junk mail, face endless amounts of advertising, and man-
handle product packaging. We're mindful of recycling (bags, plastics,
metal, etc.), we produce photos in duplicates and triplicates, and we
attend events, parties, and holiday festivities. We endure interrup-
tions and try to pay our bills.

We also drive bigger cars: four-by-four vehicles that allow us to
transport lots more stuff to our homes. Now, mind you, we don't
actually park the vehicles in our garages, because they no longer fit

into our two- or three-car garages because (ouch! here comes more . . .) the garages are full of unused treadmills and Thigh Masters, boxes of old photos still waiting to go into albums, rusted skis and poles, furniture to be repaired someday, a set of drums, two outmoded computers, and one electric typewriter, plus, well, you fill in the blanks.

We've filled our homes and garages with stuff that we don't have the time or energy to take care of! And that's not all (I know, I sound like an infomercial, right?). We're spread so thin that we have to hire housekeepers to clean our homes, trainers to exercise our bodies, bookkeepers to pay our bills, pet sitters to watch the animals, gardeners to handle the yard work, and I'm sure you can think of more examples of our topsy-turvy lifestyle. It's too much.

Even when going to the grocery store, we must be prepared to show our club card, reacquaint ourselves with which way we swipe our card through the credit card machine (and is it debit or credit?), and clearly respond to the checker asking, "Paper or plastic?" Heck, did we remember to bring our own reusable bags in from the car? Too much going on and too many choices. Let's face it. Our culture is stressing us out, which isn't really the culture's fault because we're part of it . . . so there's yet another reason we're inside a pressure cooker. What we Americans are doing in our lifetimes in response is watching fourteen to twenty-two years of television per person because we're too tired to do anything else—too tired from doing it all!

My friend and Australia's first certified professional organizing expert, Karen Koedding, was once caught up in the rat race. She decided to do something radical: she moved from America to Australia and changed her life. Here's her story:

True Confession. I'm a professional organizer and I really like my stuff. How do professional organizers learn how to organize? Are they just born that way? I don't think so; I believe that organizing is a learned life skill. It may be a passion to organize, but I think the how-to is a learned skill. I learned how to organize as a child from my parents.

When I was about seven years old my mom decided to declutter my toys and I caught her in the act. Oh no! Where was my doll going? My mom told me that she was sending it to charity. What the heck was "charity," and why was this happening? My mom explained about the "poor children"—a guilt technique used by parents around the world. Result: Me going into a complete sobbing meltdown. In that moment, that doll became my absolute favorite doll. My mom said, "You never play with it." I declared it as a terribly important doll in my life and continued crying as I held on to it with a death grip. My mom is a very smart (and loving) lady, and as we have done many times over my lifetime, we negotiated. My mom said that I needed to donate five toys, but allowed me to make the decision about which ones were to go.

This was a great life lesson: I needed to let go, there was a boundary in the quantity, and I had the power to choose. I made my selections and off the toys went. I was a smart little girl, so I made sure that I started playing with that doll. I still have that power to choose, and so do you. You have the power to choose—to keep or to let go.

Life Lesson: Decluttering and Letting Go. One day when I was about eight years old I wanted to go out and play. (Remember when kids did that?) My dad told me that I needed to clean my room before I could go out and play. I went to my bedroom and proceeded to shove a big pile of clothing and toys into the closet; shove a mass of toys into the toy box, which would not close; and shoved everything else under the bed. I thought this was very effective. After five minutes I went back to my dad and said I was done and was going out to play.

My dad said, "Wait a minute, I'm coming to inspect it first." I was quite confident he'd be impressed. He came up to my room, and then he did the unimaginable! He took my toy box and turned it upside down, dumping all of the toys on the floor. He opened the closet and pulled all of the toys and clothing out, and then he got a broom, laid down on his stomach on the floor, and pulled everything out from the under the bed. Then he said, "Now, clean up your room." Clean up my room? I just did that!

What he had done looked a thousand times worse than before I started! I was out of my mind with anger. Not only was he stopping me from going out to play, but he had made it look worse than ever. So furious! My mom told me to calm down, that she would help me. Not sure if my mom knew that my dad was going to choose that moment as life-lesson time for me, or if she had factored it into her day, but she did help me. Needless to say, I didn't get to go out and play that day, but my mom spent a few hours with me teaching me how to organize. I learned how to group like items, how to make stuff fit, and how to make the room look really nice. These are all basic organizing principles that I didn't know until I was taught them.

Life Lesson: How to Organize. When I was in my early thirties, I moved to Australia. At the time, I owned a large three-bedroom split-level house in the United States, in which I rented out three of the rooms while I was away. This allowed me to keep my stuff, which was important because I had a lot of stuff then, and I liked my stuff. I went to Australia with two small trunks and two suitcases. I was going to live there for six months. It was a major planning and organizing operation. I wanted to take everything that I may need and a bit of what I might want—a little bit of home—with me. I'd never lived away from home before. I took clothing, some office supplies, my laptop, my CDs, a few kitchen items, my teddy bear, towels, toiletries, and a few books. Once there I rented a bed and mattress, a TV, and two couches. I used one trunk as the TV stand and the other as a bed table in my bedroom. My filing system consisted of neat piles of paper on the floor, some in manila folders.

Everything else I had with me fit into my closet, the bathroom, and the kitchen cupboards. I had a great time during that (extended) seven months. I didn't have anything to take care of! I didn't have a house that I wanted to decorate. I didn't have stuff I had to dust. No stuff to move around. Very little stuff to put away. I was free! I had so much free time! I had fun! At the end of the seven months I went back to New York, knowing that I wanted to return to live in Australia again. The biggest reason was the freedom that I felt in Australia. Did this have to do with my possessions?

The next time I went to Australia, I sold my house in New York before heading Down Under. I put some of my stuff in storage in my friend's attic. I put some of my stuff in storage in my cousin's basement. I gave some of my stuff away to Goodwill. I gave some of my stuff and furniture to my family and friends. I stored some of my stuff in my mom's apartment. Whew! That was a lot of stuff! This was all exercised with a high level of organization—and stress! The stuff that I was taking to Australia fit in my two suitcases, four moving boxes, and one trunk (the other trunk had met its demise on the trip back to New York last time). I put together a list of stuff that I had donated or had given to friends/family, as I knew I might at some point wonder where my stuff had gone. I found over the next two years that I did look for a couple of things on that list, but once I knew where they had gone, it made sense to me again.

This time I was away for two and a half years. I ended up buying a few pieces of furniture and some smaller belongings. I decided to move back to New York and took my stuff with me. When I moved back to New York, for what I thought was my final big move—and a permanent one—I stayed with my cousins, along with that mound of some of my stuff in their basement. I found a place to live in

Manhattan—a one-bedroom apartment. It didn't feel right to continue to store my stuff in everyone else's homes, and I didn't want to pay for a storage unit. I had also spent the last few years living with only what I needed, so the time had come to do the big clearout. Okay, maybe the time had been a few years earlier, but I was ready now.

I cleared out my cousin's basement and my friend's attic, putting a bunch of my stuff into a garage sale, and more went again to Goodwill. I kept a grand total of about 20 percent of my stuff! Yes! Only 20 percent of my stuff! Didn't I tell you that I really liked my stuff? But now, 80 percent was gone! Guess what? I felt so much better! I still had more than enough! I narrowed down a large three-bedroom house into a small one-bedroom apartment. I had realized during those years of living without all of my stuff, plus the moving and packing and unpacking, that I didn't really need nor want all of my stuff. When I started going through my stuff in my cousin's basement and my friend's attic (stuff that I had stored as important for more than two and a half years), I didn't recognize a lot of it! I didn't even like some of it; worse, I didn't remember buying some of it, and finally, I didn't remember owning some of it.

"I'm not being a conscious spender or owner." The time and money I had spent on my stuff equaled time and money I had wasted. Looking after so much stuff was a waste of my lifetime, and I wasn't willing to do that anymore. Over the next few years I lived and worked in New York, went to school for an interior design degree, and started up my organizing firm, A Little Elf. It was a crazy, exhausting time, and I yearned for the lifestyle I had had in Australia. So guess what?

Yep! I decided to return to Australia again. This time I had a lot less stuff, but still had to declutter again. I donated some of my stuff and threw some of my other stuff out. I packed up the one-bedroom apartment and moved all of my stuff to Australia, making the full commitment to the country (and to my stuff).

I now live in a beautiful home with a view of the ocean. Everything I own fits into this apartment. I've even gotten rid of more as I moved each time. As an adult I have moved thirteen times, including five overseas moves. Each time I move I declutter and donate or throw out some of my stuff. Each time I move I want less and less to pack and unpack.

I can see correlations between clutter and poor health, unhappiness, and weight gain. When I moved to New York the last time I was heartbroken, depressed, culture-shocked, and overweight. It took me six months to unpack the final eight boxes that stared at me every day as I lay on the couch depressed. One day I made the decision to unpack those boxes, and from that point I moved forward instead of wallowing in the past. I see this all the time, when clients recover from depression or cancer, they look around at their homes and decide that they want to make a change, declutter, and get organized. Your home is truly a reflection of what is going on inside of you.

What does your stuff do for you? Is it supporting you and the life you want? Or is your stuff holding you back, giving you more to do? Is your stuff keeping you in that job you hate? Is it getting in your way of exercising and eating right? Are you working harder and more hours to support that big house with all of your stuff? Is your life going to have been worth spending on your stuff? You have the power to choose to buy or not to buy. You have the power to choose to keep or not to keep. If you're stuck holding on to your stuff, there will be clutter in your finances, your health, your job, and your personal life. Decluttering gives you strength. It gives you clarity on your priorities. It gives you time! And freedom!

Consider your spending habits. Are you like me and have bought stuff that you didn't need and only a few years later didn't want and didn't remember? Have you tried picking up that stuff that you want to buy, admiring it, and putting it back down, leaving it at the store? Tell yourself, *I'll come back for this next week and buy it.* I guarantee that for most of you, it will be out of sight, permanently out of mind, as it is only that first moment of admiring the object that provides the satisfaction. Try looking at your savings as the new beautiful stuff that you are acquiring. You'll sleep better at night. I promise. When it comes to decluttering, you will have to throw stuff out; not everything is worthy of being donated. You will have made bad purchasing decisions over your lifetime. You will have bought stuff that wasn't worth it. Don't let the stuff stay in your life. Do your part in recycling and donating, but throw the rest out. We throw out so much less than we used to forty and fifty years ago. Think about the waste the next time you go shopping; become a conscious spender and don't buy the stuff in the first place.

Think about the quality of life that you want to have. Does taking care of lots of stuff factor into that? My mom taught me the life lessons of how to declutter and organize. Over the years I've had points in my life when I've been better at it or not so good at it, but I've never forgotten the skills. Moving overseas taught me that living with less is freeing. I like that feeling. I still like my stuff a lot; I just make sure that what I keep adds to my life as opposed to draining from my life. What's more important to you: your stuff or your quality of life?

Karen's story demonstrates how even the best of us feel enslaved to our material possessions. To help you get a bit clearer on your material possessions (room by room) and the physical clutter around you and within you, try answering these questions:

Dorothy the Organizer's
Room-by-Room Clutter Quiz

Living Area

What statement best describes your living area? (Circle the answer that best applies to you.)

1. Very neat and tidy
2. Few papers lying around but other than that fine
3. Happily cluttered
4. Very messy
5. Filthy—you don't invite others over for fear of embarrassment

How would you say your friends or family describe your living area?

1. Clean.
2. Cluttered.
3. Messy.
4. It is very difficult to be around.
5. You don't invite your friends over.

Which statement best describes your thoughts about your living area?

1. You have too much stuff.
2. You're too disorganized.
3. You can't seem to part with anything.
4. Your place has grown too small for the amount of possessions you have.
5. You're immobilized by your living area.

Which statement accurately reflects your thoughts regarding your living area?

1. You are happy with it.
2. It sometimes gets to you.

3. You wish you knew where to start to clean it up.

4. You are depressed by your surroundings.

Kitchen

Let's say you don't own a dishwasher and you make a delicious dinner that uses four of your pots; you

1. Clean them as soon as you use them.

2. Clean them after dinner.

3. Clean them the next morning.

4. Clean them the next time you need to use them.

Daily Activity

After reading the daily paper, you

1. Put it in the recycle bin immediately.

2. Stack the papers to be thrown away in a few days.

3. Leave the papers where you read them.

4. Keep the papers for months.

Dining Room Table (or Office Desk)

Please complete the sentence: "I clean my dining room table [office desk] . . ."

1. Every day.

2. Once a week.

3. When it gets messy.

4. When I can't find something.

5. When my friends are coming over.

Answer Key: As you might guess, the more 4s and 5s you have circled suggest that you may need to implement some of the organizing tips in this section or even find an accountability partner to help you get organized. Remember, it's the awareness and the honesty about your situation that eventually allows you to take action.

Paper Clutter

Over the last decade I have lectured to thousands and thousands of people about clutter, and most questions seem to be about having "too much paper." One of the first articles written about my work appeared in the *Christian Science Monitor*. I was flown to Boston and reporter Mark Clayton interviewed me. As fascinating as the interview about "me" was, I was deeply intrigued when Mark offered to introduce me to one of the longstanding reporters at the paper. He called ahead to get official, secret, high-security clearance for us to visit this veteran writer. The other writer not only agreed to let me see his office, but he was proud to show me a "thing or two."

We arrived, and Mark and I and were greeted warmly. We were not, however, offered a place to sit, because, well, all the chairs were filled—with stacks and stacks of research. So was this amazing researcher's desk, floor, and credenza. Every square inch was chock-full of paper. So why would this mastermind be so proud of his paper, and even more so, why would he subject himself to what I call "the Martha Stewart experience" (you know, it's kind of like inviting Martha Stewart over for dinner and serving a takeout meal on paper plates)? But I soon learned why. All the other reporters and staff members came in to meet me while I was visiting this paper vault of an office, and each person said, "Oh yeah, Tom is our go-to guy; he knows everything! Everyone here knows that *he* will have the answer!"

"Look, I've been here ten years, and if I can't find it, I know I can go to Tom," said one staffer.

Though I was the subject being interviewed that day, I learned that stuff can represent our identity. Whether it's clothing or tools, whether it's teddy bears or foreign coins, stuff can represent our reputation to the world. Tom's reputation and his entire identity was all about being the go-to guy, the answer man, the dude at the end of the hall who knows everything. Why in the world would Tom ever want to get rid of his paper? He had the top-ranking reputation at that newspaper office, and no professional organizer in the world was going to take that away from him. I learned that lesson early, and it made a difference in my organizing career for sure.

Though Tom, the writer from the *Christian Science Monitor*, didn't want his paper touched, many people want it to flow like John Philip Sousa's marching band. Paperwork can flow readily at a steady pace, creating harmony and precision in your office and home. Author of two books, *Paper Flow* and *From Stuff to Sorted*, professional organizer MaryAnne Bennie helps clients alleviate their constant, overwhelming mountain of paperwork through some very simple but effective steps to organization. Here she gives answers to the top ten questions about paper clutter.

Top Ten Questions About Paper Clutter

After working with hundreds of clients, I have found that these top ten questions keep popping up. I have also found that once they are answered, progress is phenomenal. Take some time to read through them and apply the answers to your special situation. The answers are based on the tried-and-tested Paper Flow system, and they will become your keys to success.

1. **My house is full of piles of paperwork, and it seems like a mountain too high to climb. How and where should I start?**
   Don't despair; you are one of many people staying stuck because you may not know how to begin. Like any fresh start, you need to draw a line in the sand and separate the past from the future and focus on the now. Forgive all your past behaviors, get rid of all the blame, and give yourself a break. The best way to separate the paper past from the paper future is to box up the past. Just get as many boxes as you have piles and pack up all your

old piles into labeled boxes and stack them neatly away. *Ahhh*, you should feel better right away because the mountain is contained, labeled, and ready for when you are ready to sort them. Most important, the energy of the room will have changed, and instead of facing paper mountains, you can tackle one box or part of a box at a time.

2. **When my paperwork comes in, it ends up all over the place. What should I do?** There is a simple and obvious answer to this problem, but when you are in a muddle, nothing is obvious. All you need to do is to have a designated container placed in a logical location and from now on call it your "in-tray." Once set up, it will hold all your fresh, new, incoming paperwork, and all your other surfaces will be free of paper clutter. And remember, you have packed up the past, so you are now only dealing with the present. Feels good, doesn't it?

3. **I already have an in-tray but it just piles up to the ceiling. How do I empty it and keep it under control?** The key to success is to have a schedule to manage all of your frequent, recurring paper actions. Just like a railway system needs a timetable to keep it running smoothly, a paperwork system needs a schedule to drive it and to keep it running smoothly. All you need to do is decide how often you need to empty your in-tray on a weekly basis. Some people need to empty it daily, while others might only need to empty it once a week. The key is that you allocate time every week to completing this important task. Just think of all the time and energy you will save by tackling your in-tray on a regular basis, knowing that it will all get handled according to your schedule. Most people find this very comforting. Would you?

4. **How do I empty my in-tray? I keep procrastinating and things keep falling to the bottom and never move forward.** The key to managing your in-tray is to keep to your schedule

and to always start at the top. Once you touch a piece of paper it can never go back! Yes, paper moves out of the in-tray and moves forward into your Paper Flow system. The best way to direct paper as it leaves the in-tray is to simply ask it one critical question: "What is the very next thing I need to do with you?" The answer to that simple, but critical, question directs your paperwork onto its next station. Typically the answers are "Pay me!" "File me!" "Claim me!" "Update me!" "Reply to me!" "Read me!" So set up a Recurring Actions station with subfolders for each of these actions. Now you have a place for everything and everything in its place. The real key to success here is to not only separate your paperwork by the action that needs to be taken but also to schedule time to act on each subfile every week. For example, Bills to Pay (Monday), Claims to Make (Tuesday), Contacts to Enter (Wednesday), Items to Read (Thursday), Items to File (Friday), and Correspondence to Complete (Daily). By having one day on and six days off each of these tasks, you stay focused and in control. The beauty of Recurring Action Files is that they are your "forever files"; once set up they last you a lifetime and work hard for you every week.

5. **I have a few projects on the go and don't know what to do with the paperwork. How can I make sure I have everything I need in one place so I can get to it whenever I need to?** Project management is easy. Project files are temporary files; once a project is complete, it ceases to exist. Simply create a folder or a container to hold the amount of paperwork your project will generate. A renovation project, for example, will hold more paperwork than a party-planning project. Once your project is complete, you can clear out the file and only keep a few summary items. Some of the items that end up in your project files may also need to get processed through your Recurring Actions Files first.

www
oxyregen.com

Airdrie AB

403-502-
6477

6. **I can never find my important documents when I need them; how should I file my birth certificates, wills, passports, and other important information?** The key to important document success is to have one file dedicated to all important documents. You can use a hanging file or a display book. Simply place each document into a plastic pocket to keep it clean and wrinkle free. You can make copies to be kept with a trusted friend or with your accountant, lawyer, or bank. Many people also store backup files of important documents in the cloud so that they have access to important information wherever they are. This is especially useful in the event of an emergency situation.

7. **How long should I keep information, like bank statements, household bills, and other information for tax or budgeting purposes?** Every situation is different, so the key to success is to first check with your financial advisor about exactly what you need to keep and for how long. Then the key to success is to always have what you need on file. You could keep one year to eighteen months' worth of information in your Reference Files and then any files required after that could be moved into your Archive Files. The key to success here is to rotate your files regularly—at least once a year—to keep them flowing in, through, and out of your Paper Flow system.

8. **What is the best way to organize all my old piles? Every time I start I end up frustrated and in a bigger mess than when I started!** Remember that vertical is your friend and horizontal is the enemy. So often, people sort their big, hefty piles into smaller piles all over their horizontal surfaces. When the doorbell rings or they need their surfaces to serve dinner, it all gets packed back up into a big, hefty pile. Would it make sense to you to sort paperwork into vertical magazine boxes? If so, try this. Sort your paperwork into a series of magazine boxes and create the biggest, fattest categories you can. Like

"everything to do with banking and finance" or "everything to do with household expenses" or "everything to do with health" or "everything to do with the children." Once you have sorted all your old paperwork into these big, fat categories, you can take one at a time and subsort them into subcategories. For instance, your financial paperwork can be sorted into bank accounts, loans, and credit card accounts. The key is that all your hard work will be rewarded because during the sorting everything stays in place. You can also start and stop at any time while using as little horizontal space as possible.

9. **I do bits and pieces but really don't understand how a good paper system really flows; can you tell me how it all comes together?** Remember what we've already learned. New paperwork comes in and it goes into the in-tray. Refer to your schedule and process your paperwork by asking the critical question, "What is the very next thing I need to do with you?" The reply dictates your paperwork's next position in the system. Process each of your Recurring Action Files according to your schedule. Every week you pay your bills, make any claims due to you, reply to correspondence, update any contact details, read your reading material, and file your filing. Easy! Anything to do with projects would go into your project file until the project is complete. Every year you cull out excess files and either archive them or destroy them.

10. **It doesn't matter what I do—my in-tray and my filing always get out of control. What advice can you give me?** These two stations are the most dangerous in the system and if left unattended will obviously get out of control. Like any railway system, the schedule drives everything and your Paper Flow system is no different. You can use a few cunning strategies to keep yourself on track: rewards often work, so why not set a reward for completing the tasks you procrastinate about?

You can also play the "beat the clock" game—set a timer and see how fast you can empty your in-tray or complete your filing. You will always find it doesn't take nearly as long as you thought. If all else fails, what about outsourcing the tasks you really hate? See if another member of the family likes the tasks you don't and do a deal!

Your paperwork is evidence of who you are, what you do, and where you have been, and it provides great insight into your financial well-being. Why not make it work for you? Turn your paperwork into paperplay: make it your friend and not the enemy. Once you master your paperwork, you really will be set free. Setting it up doesn't take long, and it takes very little time to maintain. So are you ready to lose your paperweight? Are you ready to make a few changes that will radically change the way you think about and work with your paperwork?

Having a system to work with will give you a sense of control and consistency that will support you through your first few days, and once you get into the swing of it, your schedule will keep all your paperwork.

If Your Clutter Could Talk

What would your clutter say about you if it could talk? Just as the car we drive, the clothes we wear, or the color we paint our homes may suggest a bit about our personalities, so the same goes for our clutter. It could be saying a number of things to the world (and you). See if any of these examples seem familiar:

Too Much Paper

- I'm a workaholic.
- If I throw it away, I will need it again in the future and then be up a creek without a paddle.

- If I don't see it, I won't remember to do it (pay bills, submit insurance claims, write a birthday card).
- I worked years to learn all this stuff or build this business; I'm not about to throw it away!

Too Many Clothes

- I place a high value on how I look.
- I don't have a working washer and dryer.
- I've gained weight over the years and I fear letting go of the smaller clothing sizes.
- I grew up poor and always wore hand-me-downs. Now that I have some money, by golly, I'm going to buy what I want!

Too Much Food

- I can't resist a good sale and buy food in multiples.
- I always wanted to be a chef and love having lots of choices in the cupboard.
- One of my parents was an alcoholic and didn't provide me with regular meals, and I often went hungry as a child.
- I feel lonely and food seems to be my biggest and most accessible friend.

Too Many Projects

- Crafts and projects make me think of being at my late grandmother's home when I was a child. We always made something, and those times were so special to me.
- My parents wouldn't let me do anything except study. I want the freedom to create as an adult.
- I'm an artist—I need all this stuff for my inspiration.
- I started that project but somehow didn't finish and then wound up starting another.

Too Many Books

- I always wanted to write a children's book, and I just love to have kids' books around me; it feels good.
- My daughter went to live with her father when I was divorced. I've missed both of them so much that I never wanted to get rid of any of their books and bought many of my own.
- I'm interested in so many subjects. I wish I had more shelf space.
- It's a sin to throw books away.

The Beguiling Book Bartender

Pull up a stool, friends. My book-hoarding client, Meg, is ready to serve you a stiff story from her shelf of intoxicating novels and sci-fi literature. An aspiring writer by day and a bartender by night, Meg's three-bedroom apartment was floor-to-ceiling books, magazines, and newspapers. Due to the threat of an eviction from her landlord, Meg called me, and without an ounce of embarrassment, she showed me around her large and once-spacious apartment. Now, when I say Meg showed me around, I mean to say that I shimmied in through the front door, walked sideways to maneuver through the halls, and contorted my body to slide around the towers of books (which numbered nearly thirty thousand) to peer into each of her rooms.

This house of cards was ready to implode, and Meg had less than sixty days to correct her situation. My mind took snapshots of her space—a small, round, blanketed area with a pillow served as her bed . . . well, it actually *was* a bed. A California king bed. But books, multiple pairs of eyeglasses, and lamps of all sizes and shapes with burned-out light bulbs and coiled-up extension cords crowded the surface. Then there was the bathroom. The Jacuzzi bathtub served as an entire genre of mystery novels by a popular

American writer, water slowly dripping on the molded-out books below.

Meg was in utter confusion. Not because she couldn't find anything in her home, but because she could not understand why in the world her landlord was evicting her! This was her space and she wasn't hurting anyone. Books weren't dangerous! She paid her rent on time! This simply wasn't fair. Indeed, Meg's thinking was a bit distorted. She was also experiencing an unusual attachment to her books, which manifested itself as hoarding.

According to the article *Family Informants' Perceptions of Insight in Compulsive Hoarding* by David F. Tolin, Kristin E. Fitch, Randy O. Frost, and Gail Steketee, individuals with compulsive hoarding problems commonly display lack of awareness of the severity of their behavior, sometimes denying that they have a problem and often resisting intervention attempts and failing to follow through with therapeutic assignments.

Meg is not alone. Some statistics show that there are upward of 15 million people suffering from the disorder called hoarding.

Hoarding

The latest edition of the American Psychiatric Association's *Diagnostic and Statistical Manual of Mental Disorders* (*DSM*) defines a hoarding disorder as "persistent difficulty discarding or parting with possessions, regardless of their actual value." Journalist Christine Roberts of the *New York Daily News* reports, "The psychological condition made famous by reality television has long been considered a symptom of obsessive-compulsive disorder." She further reports that Randy Frost, a Smith College professor of psychology who studies hoarding issues, said the new diagnosis will ease people's "access to treatment." In other words, because this disorder is now listed in the *DSM,* more therapists, organizers, government officials, and family members will be trained to work with individuals who hoard.

Recently the producers of *Hoarders* asked me to "spend the night" in my hoarding client's home. Could I really do this? How could this possibly help the individual? In the back of my mind I was also asking the mental health question, *Is this really good for the client or is it more exploitive than I can bear? Is there truly any merit to such an experiment?*

So I thought about my own similar addiction, which I had tried to hide for years: food. I began to think about what it would be like if I had another caring human being come into my home at night to observe my eating behavior. *I hated the thought of it!* Knowing that "what we resist in life persists," I placed myself in the middle of this question and looked further to find all the uncomfortable feelings surrounding such a proposal.

Just as my hoarding clients would conduct themselves normally by day—go to work, take the kids to swim practice, go to a doctor's appointment, and so on—I would eat normally by day and especially in front of others. But at night? At home? Alone, in isolation? That's where I did my crazy food bingeing. After a late-night run to an all-night market, I would consume boxes of doughnuts, entire bags of chips, and pints of ice cream—finally falling into a sugar coma—only to awaken to the wrappers, spoons, and empty bags. Oh my Lord! *No!* I wouldn't want *anyone* to observe this behavior. If they did, I would be humiliated, and I would finally have to do something about it. Bingo! *I would finally have to do something about it.* I would have to face how I'd stuffed my face and avoided my stuff.

Had I been brave enough to talk about it, I would have saved myself a lot of personal and physical pain. This could be true for someone who drinks too much, gambles excessively, shops endlessly, smokes pot to no end, or hoards stuff to the rafters. I realized that as a professional organizing expert, I might be able to unlock the awareness for an individual who hoards by entering into their sacred nighttime ritual to observe their unusual and undiscussed behaviors. On *Hoarders* I could finally ask and see firsthand:

• Where does my client sleep when there is absolutely no bed or couch visible?
• How does an individual go to the toilet when the plumbing isn't working and the bathroom is hoarded to the ceiling?
• How can one cook for themselves or their family when the kitchen counters are full, the fridge is molding, and the stove is piled with enough mail to start a bonfire?

Yes, I knew I had the answer. I would do this. I would actually meet my hoarding client where she was—without judgment—and learn how she lives and copes in such a magnificent hoard. Perhaps I could observe and unlock for her what took me years to solve on my own. Having someone see how I operated would have required telling the truth, not just to a stranger, but to myself, too. I had worked so hard to keep that part of my life a secret (as if my carrying 200-plus pounds on my small frame wasn't obvious enough); would I really have been willing to allow someone in just to save my own life? I thought about it. *Yes. Yes, I would.*

When it comes to hoarding, my costar on *Hoarders®*, Michael A. Tompkins, PhD, and coauthor with Tamara Hartl of the book *Digging Out*, suggests implementing the "harm reduction plan" and other techniques that help us become more approachable to individuals who hoard. The harm reduction plan is a set of strategies to help people who hoard live safely and comfortably in their homes. Tompkins and Hartl explain, "A harm reduction plan identifies areas of the home or the person's behavior that specifically pose a risk to the individual. Those areas become the targets to work on. Providers and loved ones help the person who hoards manage these targets with the goal of maintaining safety and comfort." Tompkins and Hartl further explain, "In a harm reduction plan, someone visits the home of the person who hoards to assess the risks the individual faces. Maybe there is clutter on the staircase, or papers that are too close to stovetops that the loved one uses regularly. Alternatively, there are situations where the person who hoards is spending all of his or her money on acquiring new possessions yet has not paid the power or water bill. Therefore, harm reduction focuses on working with the person who hoards in a supportive and collaborative way to minimize potentially harmful behaviors like these."

Dr. Randy Frost, an internationally known expert on obsessive-compulsive disorder, compulsive hoarding, and the pathology of perfectionism, developed (along with his colleagues at Smith College) the famous OHIO Rule, which stands for Only Handle Items Once. If you handle an item, it *must* go where it belongs. *Do not* put it down to think about or decide on later. He says the decision will not get any easier by delaying it. Here are the OHIO Rule guidelines. Try them if they work for you:

- If it's broken, it goes.
- If it smells, it goes.
- If it's contaminated with bugs, mold, or animal droppings, it goes.
- Ask yourself if you have a use for it at a specific point in the future. If not, it goes.
- Are you giving it to someone on a set date in the future? If not, it goes.
- Does it have a home? If not, then it goes or something else does to give it a home.

Finally, professional organizer Christy Best, author of *Clutter's Last Stand*, also points out the correlation between a messy home and depression. She says, "Possessions, like fat, insulate us from the outside world, building a wall of junk that we can hide behind. Our clutter becomes an insular mechanism for shielding ourselves from pain. We all do this to some degree, but few ever make the correlation. The sheer act of acquiring stuff, too, can be a self-medication. How many of us shop in order to feel better? But it's a temporary fix that, in the end, only adds to our depression."

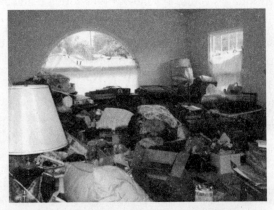

Dorothy's Client: Hoard "Before"

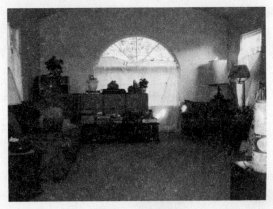

Hoard "After"

In a blog interview with Sue West, a certified professional organizing expert in New Hampshire (www.organizeNH.com), I had a chance to answer some common questions about hoarding. When you read the questions and answers, see what you can learn for yourself or someone else who hoards:

SUE WEST: What do you most enjoy in your role as lead organizer with your clients who suffer from hoarding behaviors?

DOROTHY: What I enjoy most is observing even the tiniest bit of transformation in the client; like suddenly coming to terms with a behavior pattern that has them stuck, depressed, or isolated. That realization is the key to the turning point (or not) for nearly every individual who hoards. One particular hoarding client on the *Hoarders* show was keeping *everything* from her late husband who had passed away nearly twenty years prior. She even kept an ashtray with a cigarette butt and cigarette ashes. The therapist [Dr. Suzanne Chabaud] and I asked her if this ashtray really signified her husband's life. She blinked several times like Snow White waking up after a long sleep and admitted it did not. She lifted up her head farther and saw the rest of the room, which was stuck in the year 1992, when her husband was still living. The whole show shifted and her whole life shifted. That's what I enjoy the most.

SUE WEST: With your team of professionals who work with your clients, what are a couple of the most key points you make with them?

DOROTHY: The key points I try to make with my assisting teams (or anyone who tries to help an individual who hoards) are

- You are important to me.
- Be safe while you're on the job.
- Find value for yourself in doing this work.
- Use compassion, but don't fall for any "enabling" behavior patterns with the client.

- Do not barrage the client with many questions from many people. Have a point person.
- Detach yourself from the outcome. It never turns out the way you expect it to.

SUE WEST: On the team, what other types of professions are represented?

DOROTHY: Here are just a few (there are so many):

- Therapists
- Social workers
- Clergy
- Animal control
- Prosecuting attorneys
- Veterinarians
- Child Protective Services
- Adult Protective Services
- Police
- Building and safety
- Housekeeping teams
- Painters
- Junk removal teams
- Pest control
- Hazmat cleanup crews
- Car towing services

SUE WEST: How do other organizers work with you? Most people think of organizing as working one-on-one with a client.

DOROTHY: I get résumés from organizers (and nonorganizers) who would like to work for me or my company, or be on the show. I keep a list of independent contractors whom I hire to do professional organizing work. Many of my team members have worked for my company for over ten years. When it comes to bringing in organizers to *Hoarders®*, we typically use the National Association of Professional Organizers website and input the zip code for the area in which we are filming. Those organizers who pop up in that ZIP code are usually notified of the shoot, and slots are filled on a first-come, first-served basis.

SUE WEST: When or in what instances do you call in the therapist? What issues are not for organizers or family members; where's the line?

DOROTHY: While I can give some examples, remember that there are always exceptions. In some cases, professional organizers have a PhD or have served as clinical therapists in the past. Some organizers have extensive training in the field and are not credentialed but are highly effective. In my experience, I would ask that family members or organizers who are working with an individual who hoards seek guidance if:

- The client has spoken of suicide.
- The client is hoarding animals and the animals are clearly neglected.
- The client is facing criminal charges or eviction, or Child Protective Services is involved.
- The client is using/abusing substances.
- The client has no support system whatsoever (family, friends, social worker).
- Young children are involved and they are neglected.

Tackle Clutter: Organizing Systems and Habits for Success

Oh, no, here it is—the truth about me: I am a type-A personality. That's probably why I'm a professional organizer. I've got so many darn tips on the subject of clutter, I just had to find a way that is super-duper easy for you to find what you need when you need it. The best approach? A to Z. If kindergartners can operate using this system, so can I! Listed below are tips for organizing your clutter in a quick A-to-Z format. So, if you want a tip for your key chain, go to "K." If you want a tip to reduce magazine clutter, go to "M."

Can't find it what you're looking for in my list? E-mail me at info@ DorothyTheOrganizer.com. I've got you covered.

A

Addresses or Contact Info

1. Gather all business cards and small slips of papers with addresses and phone numbers from around the house or the office.
2. Once bunched together, sort the enormous pile into alphabetical piles.
3. Rubber band all the "A" contacts, "B" contacts, "C" contacts, and so on.
4. Enlist help to have the cards scanned or typed into your contact list or written into your address book.

Artwork

If you are a parent of a preschooler, you know all about the outrageous volume of artwork that comes home from school—all of it meant to be saved forever! I suggest putting a cap on the amount of artwork. For example, for this school year, find one bin in which to store your young Picasso's work. All incoming work goes into the bin. When the bin is full, it's time to do a quick review. Pick out one or two of your favorite pieces and keep those. Then, ask your child to pick out their favorite two pieces, and—gulp—toss the rest. Believe me, more and better artwork will come right back in the door tomorrow afternoon!

B

Baskets

Rather than looking for ways to store and organize your existing baskets, which take up space, why not use these multipurpose weaves of art to store other items? *Ba-boom*—two or three space dilemmas handled in one fell swoop. Use baskets for remote controls, gloves, mail, magazines, toilet paper rolls, hand towels, bread baskets, CD storage, makeup, belts, scarves—*ay, caramba*! Point is, if you've got the baskets hanging around anyway, put them to work until you really need them again.

C

CDs and DVDs

1. Gather all of your discs into one area.
2. Open each to confirm each disk is in the correct jewel case.
3. Get a shelf or a box large enough for all of your discs and future discs to fit.
4. Put them in an order of your choice (alphabetical or by category).
5. Keep them near your music or entertainment center for easy playing.
6. When you are done playing a disc, return it to its place.
7. Consider switching to the cloud and keeping all your music or videos there.

Closets

If you're the type of person who drapes your clothing over chairs or tosses items on the floor, it is not likely you'll have the interest or motivation to neatly hang your clothes on hangers each and every night (same goes for kids, too). Avoid purchasing newfangled, space-saving hangers that will scream at you from the back of the closet for not being used again today. Instead, install eight to ten hooks in your closet and hang clothing on them. While this is not the *perfect* answer, your clothes have a better chance of staying off the floor. The point is to create an easy system that you or your kids can maintain.

D

Desk

1. If your intention is to organize the desk, you must focus on that task only (not file drawers, supply shelves, or return e-mails). Organize the desk.
2. Enroll a colleague's or family member's help and agree on the amount of time you will spend on this project and set a timer.
3. Collect all the papers from all over the desk and make just one pile.
4. Begin sorting that huge stack of papers into categories (don't sign anything, don't flip through a journal), just sort by category—bills with bills, kids' artwork with kids' artwork.
5. Decide which of the piles is most important.
6. Make an appointment with yourself (in your calendar) to work on the important pile.

E

Earrings, Bracelets, and Other Jewelry

1. Gather up all your jewels from the bedroom, bathroom, and kitchen windowsill.
2. Lay out a white pillowcase or cotton dishcloth.
3. Empty all of your dazzling bits out in front of you.
4. Pull out any tarnished, broken, or mismatched pieces, and then decide what to keep, sell, or give away. With whatever's left, consider sorting by color (suggestions include silver, gold, by gem color, or pearl color). If you're looking for a new way other than the traditional "rings with rings" approach, perhaps storing by color will make organizing and accessorizing more fun!

F

Filing

It's time to come clean, folks. When it comes to paper and filing, are you a piler and a stacker or a filer? In my seminars, nearly 98 percent of hands go up when I ask the question, "How many of you seem to just stack your paper rather than file it?" Such an overwhelming response suggests that we need to create a system for the people rather than force the people into a system. Therefore, it is my recommendation to take a bookshelf and use it as a "pile system" rather than creating a file system in a drawer.

1. Create broad, easy categories: Bills to Pay, Kids' School Stuff, Food Program Paperwork, and Newsletters and Catalogs I Want to Read.
2. Stack your neat paper categories on the shelves (you can use decorative bins and baskets too).
3. Attach a sticky note on the shelves near each paper pile, noting the category.
4. Just do the basics—get the papers off your desk, the kitchen counter, or dining room table and onto the proper pile on your bookshelves. At the end of the year, toss what you don't need and box up that year's worth of piles. Start all over again.

G

Gifts

Birthdays, Mother's Day, Hanukkah, Christmas, going-away parties, and graduations are all cause for gift giving. But gift giving does not, however, mean gift keeping. Remember, you don't need to keep something just because it's a gift. After a big event (especially for little kids), it's important to go through the gifts you've received and decide what to do with them. Will you keep them, regift, return, or perhaps donate them? If you're given a new book and you know you won't read it, do not store it with your other books. Put the book by the doorway going out of the house with the gift receipt taped to it to be exchanged. Regifting it is an option as well. You want to stop the incoming clutter before it even starts—don't mix it with your existing stuff or that item will never see its way out the door.

H

Heirlooms

1. Unless you are using them or already displaying them, bring all heirlooms together in one room (if possible).
2. Sort like items with like items.
3. Ask yourself the story behind each "collection." If it's a meaningful piece or collection, keep it! If not, and you feel an obligation to keep it anyway, consider taking a photo of yourself and the family with the heirloom and frame the memory and let the piece or the collection go.

I

Important Documents

So, you want to know how long to keep important documents? Here is a general guideline (but always check with your doctor, accountant, or attorney for special circumstances):

Bank statements and credit card records: Keep only if there is a possible tax issue—and then you only need to keep for six years. Keep CD info until they've matured. If your bank statement doesn't contain anything you need for your taxes, you can shred immediately.

Car or homeowner's insurance: Hold on to these for approximately four years after the policy expires or until you get a new one in the mail.

Estate materials: Keep wills and trusts indefinitely. In fact, keep an extra copy and put the original in a safe-deposit box.

Health records: Keep records of kids' immunizations and your kids' and your own hospital records indefinitely, especially if you have had an abnormality or special medical experience, such as cancer, bypass surgery, and so on.

Investment and retirement account statements: Many of these are cumulative, so your year-to-date activity is usually noted on each statement. Thus, there is no reason to keep old statements. I suggest keeping annual summaries, even though you can access them electronically.

Official government documents such as birth or death certificates, passports, divorce or custody agreements, and Social Security cards: Keep, keep, keep. Better yet, in a safe-deposit box or home safe.

Paid bills: Keep them one year at best. Use the information to reconcile your taxes each year and shred. Keep important bill payments in your "tax backup folder."

Pension plan information: Keep this information indefinitely, whether it's from a current or former employer.

Property records: Documents such as mortgage applications, deeds, and loan agreements should be kept for as long as you own the property. Always save proof of loan payoffs indefinitely.

School transcripts, diplomas, and report cards: Keep transcripts if you have an inkling that you'll seek further education. Keep diplomas indefinitely. Report cards are considered memorabilia and there's usually no practical reason to keep them.

Warranties, guarantees, and manuals: Keep these booklets for as long as you own the item. Keep them all together in one place and make it a regular practice every couple of years to review the file and toss what's no longer relevant.

J

Junk Drawer

1. Locate your junk drawer; most of us have one (you know . . . the middle drawer in your desk or in the kitchen, the farthest drawer from the stove, etc.). It has random items: rubber bands, bread twist ties, loose change, old Super Glue, a screwdriver, out-of-date stamps, mismatched caps from pens and markers. . . .
2. Take an old white towel and place it on the dining room table or counter.
3. Dump the entire contents of the drawer.
4. Sort like with like (resist the urge to toss or match a lost item with its mate). Just sort: credit cards with credit cards, business cards and little pieces of paper with addresses together, paper clips together, lip glosses, nail files, and other small toiletry items together.
5. Take the "grouped like items" to their proper location: paper clips back to the desk. Lip glosses back to the makeup bag, extra coins to the kid's piggy bank.
6. Decide if you really need a junk drawer. If not, decide what would work better for you in the drawer. If you do want to keep the junk drawer, put the scissors, screwdriver, tape, bag twist ties, and old stamps back in the drawer and make a note in your calendar to clean the junk drawer again in eight months.

K

Keys

Maintain one spot for all keys in the house and put them in the same place every time. It may be helpful to label all the keys for your household such as "garage," "pool gate," "van." Also, if you consider color coding your keys, it can make them much easier to find when you're rushing about.

L

Luggage and Other Bags

I'm not sure why, but my clients love their bags and suitcases. It seems there is a bag for every purpose these days, and many of us feel the need to own all those crafty carry cases. Owning and using these travel monsters can be a bit scary. The question here is do you use each and every one of them? My guidelines are a bit strict on this one, simply because luggage and bags in general are space guzzlers.

- If the luggage is in disrepair, consider letting it go.
- If you have the same size of any piece, send it out.
- If you don't really use the item much, but feel a strong attachment to it, try using it as a storage container for other items around the house or store the luggage in a less "exclusive" place than your bedroom closet, so it doesn't steal your valuable space, which is close to you.
- Nest your bags, one inside the next, purses, laptop cases, all-purpose carry bags.

M

Magazines

1. Collect magazines from all over the house, car, and office.
2. Sort like subscriptions together.
3. Place the cooking magazines in the kitchen, travel magazines in the bedroom, and the welding and DIY magazines at the workbench.
4. Set a time boundary for yourself; if you don't read your magazines within three months, give them to the local hospital.

Memorabilia

1. Collect all memorabilia from all parts of the house and office.
2. Sort memorabilia by person or event.
3. Ask yourself what the story is behind each piece. If it is truly meaningful, prepare to store it or display it.
4. Designate a memorabilia section in your home or office that is clean and dry.
5. Store memorabilia in protective containers in designated areas.

N

Nail Files, Combs, and Toothbrushes

Your bathroom can be an organizational dream or a downright disaster. If you prefer an easy-access situation and you need a bit more organizing space, you might consider the following: Purchase a plastic three-drawer storage container that will fit under your bathroom sink. Pick the categories that are most important to you and divide your toiletries into three categories: Hair, Teeth, and Nails. Label the drawers. In the Hair drawer, store your combs, brushes, clips, and hair bands. In the Teeth drawer, store your floss, toothpaste, toothbrushes, and dental guards. In the Nails drawer, store your files, clippers, polish removers, and polishes. You can make a drawer for medications or one for cosmetics. When you need something from the drawer, it pulls out easily and goes right back.

For bigger items like deodorant, soaps, and hair sprays, use the medicine cabinet or purchase a spinning lazy Susan meant for the kitchen and place it under the bathroom sink. You won't have to get down on your hands and knees to see what you've got—just spin the wheel and you've found your fortune!

O

Office Supplies

This is one category where folks repeatedly overspend. The allure of organizational product promises and the new release of a pack of Day-Glo color gel pens is all it might take to break us down. The real tip here? Avoid buying the stuff to begin with. If you do have supplies to organize, I like a rolling plastic cart with lots of drawers that can be stored neatly under a desk or used as a table for your mouse and pad. Try six drawers and designate each drawer with its like-minded sisters and brothers—and remember to take a regular inventory. When you are able to glance into each drawer, you'll know what you need.

Drawer No. 1   Pens, pencils, markers

Drawer No. 2   Sticky notes, note pads, labels

Drawer No. 3   Checkbooks, stamps, petty cash

Drawer No. 4   Small electronics (calculators, flash drives, printer cartridges)

Drawer No. 5   Tape, glue sticks, scissor, three-hole punch

Drawer No. 6   Note cards, envelopes

P/Q

Photographs

1. Gather your photographs from all over the house.
2. Decide how you like to look at photos (computer, albums, individually).
3. Group your photos into categories like people or events.
4. Set an appointment time for yourself to either scan, create albums, or lovingly toss all of them into an old suitcase for easy retrieval.
5. Digital photo organization requires coming up with general categories for easy access. Examples are: Family, Trips, Holidays, Nostalgia, Friends.

R

Remote Controls

How often do you experience complete frustration when you can't find the darn remote control? The solution: keep a "home" for the remotes and make sure all family members know where to return them every time. Something as simple as labeling each remote (for the TV, DVD player, or stereo) and then storing them together in one decorative basket does the trick.

S

Spices

Forgive me, Julia Roberts (remember the movie *Sleeping with the Enemy*, where she was required to have all food labels in the pantry facing forward?). You do not need to do this! When it comes to organizing your spices, ask yourself if you're really a kitchen aficionado. Do you cook a lot and use spices, or do you tend to purchase a lot of premade foods? If you and your sweetie aren't doing much cooking, then lose the fancy spice rack on the counter. Eliminate that clutter and save the space for something that really matters.

If you do like to use spices, make sure they are in arm's reach of the cook. Many of us use a cupboard near the stove, but you can also use a drawer as well. Many companies make spice dividers for drawers, and this method keeps spices away from the heat of the stove, prevents bottles from being knocked over, and it's much easier to read the labels (even if they are facing out, Julia).

T

Toys

Encourage all your family members to clean up after themselves (even toddlers) by creating a "home" for their toys and items. Using pictures on the outside of a bin can help your child understand where to put dolls versus cars. For those of you who have school-age children, it will be helpful to teach them to put away toys and then gather their school items the night before (such as their backpacks with all their essential items already zipped up). Then put the backpack in the same location each and every time to eliminate last-minute scrambling.

U

Underwear and Socks

When it comes to socks, a big complaint is "stretched out elastic." To preserve the sock, avoid rolling up one sock and then fitting it over the top of the other one—socks don't like that! Unless you have a serious "thing" for socks—no kidding—pick a drawer and toss them all in (perhaps divided by color). Eliminate the time-consuming matching process at the front end, and if you put a cap on the number of socks in the drawer, matching them up when dressing will be a cinch, too.

Undies? This one's just for the gals. If you want to keep your bras in excellent shape, clip them onto skirt hangers and hang them in the closet. Avoid folding one cup inside the other; brassieres are expensive, and you don't want them to lose their elasticity before their time!

V

Videos

Online video storage is great for backup, memory preservation, and so on. If you go this route, be sure to have a system to organize, search, find, and view your favorite home videos, so that whether you're looking back on your kid's high school graduation from six years ago or splicing your child's sixteenth birthday party with his or her sixth birthday party, it's important to make sure this process is easy. Having your personal videos organized for you in a single place makes enjoying those memories even easier. Whether you decide to organize your videos online or physically or both, be sure you keep the systems uniform. By that, I mean that if you organize your videos online chronologically, do the same in your physical world. Keeping the digital world parallel to your physical world definitely makes your life easier.

W–Z

Wardrobe

My favorite organizing tip must come out of the closet now. If you want to *organize your clothes* in your closet, that's just great, but what I love to do is *organize the outfits* in the closet. This is one fun and amazing project: you will need a friend or two, a few cups of tea, and a camera. Ladies and gentlemen, slide open the closet doors and get creative. This tip is not about organizing short sleeves with short sleeves, it's all about trying on outfits, deciding what you like, and taking a photograph of yourself in the outfit. Make a pact to create at least seven to fourteen outfits with the clothes that are in your closet. Use your scarves and jewelry to accessorize and snap the photo. Capture the look and keep it on a bulletin board in your closet. This is as time-efficient and as ready-to-go as you can get. Once the pictures are posted, there is no more thinking required in the early-morning hours.

4

BANISH YOUR EMOTIONAL CLUTTER:
Learning Emotional Resistance

Face Your Failures

Landmark Education offers a fantastic course to its gradu-
ates called "Exploring a Fulfilled Life." Nice title for a
course being held at the elegant Spanish Mission–style
inn that boasts an enviable location atop an ancient thermal mineral spring flowing from 1,100 feet below and historically
revered by Native American tribes for its healing power.

The swanky Fairmont Resort and Spa in Sonoma, California,
offered me grape seed scrubs, nurturing Watsu (floating massages in
thermal water), and Chardonnay olive oil sugar polishes and exfo-
liation treatments (did someone say sugar?). Landmark Education

arranged for candlelit dinners in the bowels of an old winery, tastings, and descriptions of each meal course with its selected wine pairings to sample over hours of philosophical discussion. Yet, a day and half into the retreat, I realized I was in a week-long workshop affectionately referred to as "The Failure Course." *Noooo, no, no, I wasn't, girl. I wanted success, you people, success! What is this malarkey, studying my failures? Get me outta here!*

I thought I was in the wrong place, but in reality I was in the right place at the right time. I gave this "failure stuff" some deep thought during one of my meditation sessions and remembered that even Tom Peters, one of my business gurus, in his book *Re-Imagine!* speaks of "failing your way to the top." Okay. Maybe I could do this. I mean, what's the big reaction here? I'm just studying my past failures so that I can self-correct and move forward. Yes, I could use this information. Yes, my clients would benefit. The next morning, I sat on the edge of my chair.

The transformation started to take hold immediately. I learned that to get something valuable out of my failures, I needed to

- Just look at the facts.
- Take out all the stories and the justifications and explanations.
- With what's left, ask what I can learn from this.

Finally, I stopped all of my complaining. I stopped repeating the same, lengthy, over-detailed, drawn-out stories, and I simply said:

- I was a gymnast. I had negative thoughts. I fell off the balance beam. I came in third place.
- I stopped talking about how I came from a small town and we had subpar gym equipment to practice on, that I had a stomachache the night before, and that other gymnasts got more warm-up time than I did.
- I looked at the facts that were left and said: I had a negative

thought and image. It caused me to lose an important competition. I have learned that I can only surround myself with positive thoughts and people, especially at crucial moments in my life.

Ba-da-bing, ba-da-boom. Failure complete. I repeated the same steps regarding my failure to listen to my intuition, workaholic choices, relationships, and more. Yeah, I explored a fulfilled life. Good title for a course!

Face Your Fears and Anxieties

The Lioness of Laundry

Have you ever had so much laundry that it started piling up outside of the basket and began cascading onto the floor? How about into the whole next bedroom? Perhaps even into the living room? And a bit into the kitchen? Indeed that's what happened to my client Amy. In fact, she had so many clothes and so much laundry, she wore her washing machine out . . . and she also could no longer *get* to the washing machine—way too much stuff in the way, you see.

Amy bought more and more clothes each week because she said she could never find the clothes she had or they were never clean. Therefore, Amy invested in a kiddy pool and some laundry soap and did her wash outside on the lawn. Piles upon piles of clothes towered so high, you could have played "king of the hill" with the neighborhood kids. In the winter months the wet clothing took on a frozen sculpture look due to the melting snow by day and below freezing temperatures by night. Yes, she took care to sort the whites with whites, delicates with delicates, and color-blended clothes with color-blended clothes, of course. But the piles became taller than Amy, and her neighbors called the city health department. Amy was in trouble.

As it turned out, the reason for Amy's hoarding was fear. Her washing machine broke down, and she didn't want to let anyone into her already overpacked home to fix it. Living alone and not wanting to tell her only living brother about her situation, Amy began washing her clothes in the bathtub. Somehow, the tub overflowed, a leak had sprung, and then none of the plumbing in the bathroom worked at all. Being a bit of a "do-it-yourselfer," Amy shut off the water to the house and began using the garden hose outside to wash her clothes and handle "other business." With each new plateau, Amy's fear grew and so did her piles of clothes. If she couldn't wash them, she would just keep buying more.

In an effort to save Amy from her complaining neighbors and looming public health officials, she and I began working together to allay her fears. First we called the neighbors and public health office to apologize and communicate how we were going to get the backyard clear. Her anxiety lessened. Next, we called Amy's brother to tell him the truth about her situation and then enlist his help in repairing the plumbing. Her fears were diminishing. From there, we sorted through clothes—for days. Little by little they were categorized: keep, throw away, give away—and Amy was hopeful. It wasn't just with the hoarding that Amy needed help; she really needed help facing her fears.

I had faced a few fears of my own. One day shortly after I moved to California, the residents of Los Angeles woke up to one of the worst earthquakes it had experienced in recent history. Asleep in the dark of night, this Midwestern girl, who only knew tornadoes, found herself in her bed, which felt like being in a boat keeling from side to side due to rousing waves and wind. The sound of breaking glass surrounded me, and the only light I could see were fires in the distance. I did not know what was happening until people with flashlights gathered outside my apartment windows screaming, "Earthquake!"

With sizable aftershocks coming every few minutes, I felt my back stiffen just like it does when a police car starts following me (and I'm not even speeding). That fight-or-flight response took over, and my inner alarm was turned on for good. This disaster brought my dearest friends, Jeanette and Kevin, into my life—two people who would not only help me through the natural disaster in this moment but the man-made disasters yet to come.

So frightened. What to do? Eat.

A week after the powerful 6.8 magnitude earthquake, we were still scooping buckets of water from the apartment complex swimming pools to heat water for dishes and bathing, and I found myself returning from a business trip on the East Coast. The pilot announced we were "experiencing noxious fumes in the cabin." A lover of flying and an adventurer, I was suddenly paralyzed with fear. I asked a complete stranger to hold my hand while the oxygen masks dropped and we prepared for disaster (well, at least in my overactive mind).

We eventually landed in Las Vegas—it was a small problem with the plane's engine—and we were told we would be flying home on a different aircraft. Sure, *they* might be flying home, but not me! Would I rent a car and drive the four hours from Vegas to Los Angeles? How about a bus or the train? There was no time; I had to decide another option or board the new plane. I chose to fly, and I promised this would be the last flight I would ever take again in my lifetime.

So alarming. What to do? Eat.

Some days later, the newest and biggest fear presented itself. I've never ever known panic attacks. Heard about them, but I'd never experienced them. Suddenly, I began having a fear of going to sleep at night, a fear of driving in heavy traffic, a fear of elevators, a fear of bridges, or even fear of visiting a friend whose house was located farther than five miles from a hospital. Yep, full-blown agoraphobia! What was happening to me? First, I'd never be able to fly again, because of the whole noxious fumes incident—I resigned myself to train trips and RVing—and now this?

It seemed the only fear I didn't have was opening another pack of chocolate chip cookies. I had *never* been afraid of anything, except maybe the high dive at the local pool in my hometown. What happened to me? For months, I made multiple trips to the ER, just positive that I was having a heart attack; after all, my dad passed away from complications of a heart attack. Nope. Full-blown, life-changing, angry-making panic attacks. What was happening to me?

So disappointing. What to do? Eat.

Really, could it get any worse? Well, of course! I was expecting it to! I was beginning to find the evidence in my daily living to support how bad my life was. The more evidence I unearthed, the bigger the reason I had to retreat to the world of comfort food. The truth of the matter is that we have great experiences and not-so-great experiences every day, interspersed with magical moments and dismal dilemmas. I just couldn't see that.

While working at the UCLA School of Public Health, not only did I have the great opportunity to work for the dean as his executive assistant, but I was also responsible for a staff member, Sam, who carried out all of the building management tasks. Faculty members were locked out of their offices? Sam was there with the magic key and a smile. The elegant water fountain symbolizing health and life wasn't working at the front entrance to the building? Sam quietly fixed it. Too many students hanging outside, blowing smoke and dropping cigarette butts right in front of our building sign (which said "School of Public Health"—"public health" being the key words here) Sam ushered them gently away. Sam Lucas had been at UCLA's School of Public Health for thirty years, and everyone knew him and loved him.

So, on top of the earthquake, followed by an alarming airplane ride, which opened up painful panic attacks, here came the next one: our Sam had developed the rare and deadly "flesh-eating virus." Sam had no family, and my dear friend Diana and I were asked to sign on as Sam's "next of kin" to make the most dreadful decisions about his life and death.

A week later Sam died. Diana and I put together a memorial service for Sam that drew attendees you'd expect at the funeral of a U.S. president. Deans, high-ranking professors, colleagues, hospital administrators, and students who had known Sam came to pay him their respects.

I was tired. What to do? Eat.

That part of my life was a blur. I've since learned in my program that whenever you're in the depths of your addiction, you lose clarity. I lost clarity. I lost connection. I didn't keep up my relationships, and I isolated with my favorite food stash each night. Come to think of it, my husband was traveling a lot—it was just me and my food. The only way I could think to soothe myself was to eat in secret alone. Things couldn't get any worse, could they? (Come on, you just know what's coming, don't you?) Two nights after Sam died, I called my hubby to ask how his trip to Seattle was going. He didn't answer his cell phone or hotel room phone. I remember Bob telling me how he was going out for special Copper River salmon and he might be back late, so I really shouldn't bother to call him.

But I did call. I called every hour on the hour until midnight! I was grieving, having anxiety attacks, and needed to talk to someone other than the food. The someone I spoke to, however, was a police officer. The hotel manager had checked my husband's room to find that he had one pair of shoes, some business papers, and his wedding band piled on the desk in his room. The rest of his stuff? Apparently, it was *with him* at another woman's home (we'll just call her Copper River Salmon Sally). Okay, I fully understood what Bob meant when he said, "I'm going out for special Copper River salmon and won't be home until late." The police had located Bob's car, and indeed he was staying with Copper River Salmon Sally.

The next day and one pint of ice cream later, Bob returned my calls asking *me* what was wrong? I did the usual thing: "Where were you last night? I couldn't reach you. What happened?" He did his usual thing: "What, me? I was there; I just got back to the hotel room early and took my phone off the hook so I could get some sleep." I sat there holding the phone. This was total "BS" and I had proof!

For the first time something clicked for me. I stopped engaging in the talk and I took some liberating action. It would be a long time before I would actually extract myself from this unhealthy relationship, but there's always a point in time in which we finally "get it" and want to do something about it. Here's what I did.

I didn't mention to Bob that I knew where he really was the night before. I didn't ask any more questions. I finished the phone call calmly, and we hung up. Bob was due home the next day, and I was due to start dialing some numbers of my own:

1. Call the credit card companies. All the credit cards were in my name, and I had Bob immediately removed from the cards with no spending privileges.
2. Call the bank. The ATM card was linked to the joint checking account we shared. I moved all the cash.
3. Call our cell phone carrier. I paid all the bills and I had his phone turned off.
4. Call the locksmith. I changed the locks on the doors.
5. Call a therapist.

The next day I received a collect call from Bob—very confused and aggravated—no, I would say pissed off. A few minutes into our conversation, he realized I knew what he had done, and he became deeply apologetic about his actions from the night before. (I mean, really, what were his options?) How was he supposed to return and pay for his car rental and pay for and pick up his own car at the parking garage when he got into Los Angeles? How could he call his boss? How could he get into the house? (Well, honey, I guess you should have thought about that before you decided not to clean your room.) Ah yes! This "mysterious older man" was turning back into his sixteen-year-old immature self. For a fleeting moment, I had the guts to take action regarding this deceitful marriage and take care of myself.

This was also the beginning of my understanding about how I was not "facing my stuff" about my marriage, though I hadn't yet connected the "stuffing my face" formula into the equation. My default mode, even during therapy, was to quell my anxiousness and pain with food, interspersed with manic and momentarily successful diets. I guess if I wanted to really get out of this marriage, something extreme would have to happen—like going to jail! I didn't. But as you know, Bob did. But even then, the consequences of my not facing my stuff continued for years.

Current Research on Failures, Fears, and Anxieties

My esteemed colleague Gillian Drake watched me suffer and break through my fears and failures. After reading Dr. Carl Beuke's article in *Psychology Today* (October 19, 2011), she summarized his work and asked the question: Are we simply high achievers or failure avoiders? Here's the scoop:

> Current psychological research shows that "success" results are not as dependent upon our intellect and abilities as we might think. There's a reason why motivational speakers are so highly respected and sought after. It's not so surprising that motivational drive is a key factor in high achievers, but what is somewhat intriguing is what

those who are less successful are motivated by. Rather than being motivated by accomplishment and gratification, individuals who achieve less are motivated by the fear of failure: instead of playing to win, they are playing not to lose.

So how do the two different mind-sets impact overall results? High achievers are motivated to accomplish, consequently eager and willing to put forth intense effort over an extended period of time in the pursuit of their goals, doing whatever it takes. This includes planning the necessary steps, researching or learning necessary information they need, and exhibiting can-do, rise-to-the-challenge, whatever-it-takes-to-get-the-job-done, and won't-be-defeated attitudes.

Alternatively, people who are motivated "not to fail" are only focused on protecting themselves from embarrassment and saving "face" in front of others because they fear only mediocre results. As a result they approach their goals from a less logical perspective, allowing themselves to feel overwhelmed, focusing on the negative, fearing that they may not make the grade, and worrying about what others will think if they are not perfect. If avoidance is not possible, they are less likely to even begin planning and do not actuate the necessary steps to complete tasks, often adopting procrastination or self-sabotaging behavior (e.g., a late night over-drinking before an important morning meeting). Also, they may just give up when the going gets rough or if success and positive results are not readily forthcoming.

Both types exist on either end of the teeter-totter, with most of us falling somewhere in between. Where you fall in the balance is called "Relative Motive Strength," which depends on a number of key factors or self-beliefs. Our Relative Motive Strength does not exist in a vacuum but is calibrated by an intricate maze of beliefs that justify the commitment of intense effort toward goal achievement, or the relative lack thereof.

Here are a few questions that might indicate more prevalent failure-avoidant behavior:

- Have you rejected opportunities because you thought you were not qualified enough?
- Do you downplay your abilities because you don't want to appear arrogant?
- Have you jeopardized your chances for success because of limiting self-talk and beliefs?
- Have you procrastinated and missed deadlines because your efforts were not yet perfect?
- Do you try to do everything yourself instead of paying for help so you can focus on your true talent?
- Are you an overachiever, taking on too much or failing to prioritize, which causes underperformance or poor task completion?

1. **Who's Responsible for Success?** More highly motivated achievers tend to believe that effort, initiative, and persistence are key factors in determining the success or completion of tasks and goals. But Failure Avoiders are more likely to believe that their success depends on available resources or constraints imposed (e.g., the task is too hard or the marker was biased).

2. **Opportunities or Pitfalls?** Achievement-motivated folks tend to see challenging tasks where success is uncertain as opportunities, adopting a positive attitude of "anything worthwhile is difficult, so stop acting so surprised." Failure-avoiding folks are more likely to see pitfalls or "threats" that may lead to embarrassment or failure.

3. **Commitment to Excellence or Overwhelmed by Stress?** More highly motivated achievers tend to think of intense efforts put forth to complete demanding tasks as dedication, commitment, concentration, and involvement; they feel that hard work is necessary to get desired results. But Failure Avoiders feel that such efforts are overwhelming or stressful;

they feel persistence despite setbacks and obstacles is slightly compulsive.

4. **Valuable Life Lessons or Missing Out on Life?** Achievement-motivated folks tend to actually enjoy hard work and value learning experiences. Failure Avoiders may mock or shy away from hard work, thinking it uncool, stressful, or a waste of time, preferring to play, socialize, seize the day, and live life to the fullest.

5. **Growing and Evolving or Playing the Hand You Were Dealt?** More highly motivated achievers tend to believe that they can improve their skill sets and performance, embracing training or coaching and practicing patience and dedication to learning. But Failure Avoiders feel that they have innate talents or skills that they were born with and their ability to perform or achieve is dependent upon them.

6. **If at First You Don't Succeed, or I Screwed It Up, or I Just Don't Know How?** Achievement-motivated folks tend to believe that continued effort and commitment will overcome initial obstacles or failures. "You have to knock on 100 doors before you get one positive response." But Failure Avoiders tend to see initial failure as a sign of things to come. "Why keep banging your head against a brick wall?"

The beliefs held by more highly motivated achievers are not necessarily more logical or objectively correct than the beliefs held by Failure Avoiders—certainly not in all situations. However, they are empirically associated with high levels of achievement. Once you understand the different attitudes and beliefs of achievement-motivated versus failure-avoiding actions and thinking, you will recognize them when you hear others talk about their goals, dreams, successes, and setbacks. You will also recognize them in your own thinking and actions, and you can choose to cultivate the beliefs and steps that will support you to achieve your goals.

Organizing Tips for Failures, Fears, and Anxieties

To assist you in overcoming your fears and failures, I am sharing the script I utilized to face down my fear of flying. I got this idea from the book *Flying Without Fear* by Dr. Duane Brown. Just like I buckled down to learn and experiment with any other self-help book I bought, I read this one from cover to cover. If Dr. Brown suggested that I wear rubber bands on my hands while flying and snap them to interrupt my negative and fearful thoughts during turbulence, I did it. If he suggested I interview a pilot to see how he felt about flying a plane safely, I did it! If he told me that many pilots keep a picture of their wives and kids in the rim of their uniform hat, I would ask to see them. If Dr. Brown suggested I make an appointment with air traffic control at LAX to banish my fear of flying, I was on the phone. I learned that turbulence is sometimes like driving on a bumpy ol' back road—not all roads are paved perfectly, and sometimes you hit a few pebbles and sometimes you hit a few potholes. Yeah, it made sense. I was no longer going to stuff my face over this fear and perceived failure. I started facing my stuff!

If you have any fear you want to bust up and smash to pieces, I suggest using my script as a guide, and write one that is similar but that applies directly to your situation. I have used this method with my friend Anita, who was fearful of having brain surgery; my friend Ruth, who is afraid of dogs; and myself, when I sat down to write this book. If you write a mantra that counters your fears and you read it every night before you sleep, something happens. It's like your brain takes in the new information and creates newer, more positive, and more helpful neural pathways in your brain.

Dorothy's Script for Overcoming Fear of Flying (Concept Can Be Applied to Any Fear)

If you are facing any fear, anxiety, or phobia, you might consider reworking my notes below to accommodate your situation. By using this method, I retrained my brain to believe I would be safe while flying and could manage my anxiety. I have since used this type of script to overcome my early fears of speaking in public and managing myself in important meetings.

- I sleep exceedingly well knowing that I'm going to fly.
- I am excited to conquer my fear and become confident again. I'll need it when I travel the world for my business and television engagements and motivational speaking engagements all over the world.
- I am gaining control of something I've been afraid of, just like elevators and subways and boats. I conquer them all. I am a master at working it through. I read so many books on this. I am most capable. I have overcome hiking for hours at high altitudes, cruising in the ocean during high waves, suspension bridges, trams, and tunnels, too.
- Remember, I will have a better image of myself. Others will be proud of me. No more disappointments in myself. I will also get to see family and go to parts of the world I still yearn to see. So far, I've flown alone, in bad weather, to Wisconsin and San Francisco several times. I'm scheduled to go to Alaska, Arizona, and now Colorado—then Boston and perhaps Florida, too. I see myself flying successfully and without anxiety. Plus, I will gain more time. I am calm and relaxed when I fly. This is my new area of success.
- I've already made fantastic strides, beginning with buying and reading Dr. Brown's *Flying Without Fear*, doing the exercises faithfully, discussing the book, listening to my "overcoming

fears" tape, and visiting the airport control tower. These are all reasons to be proud of myself. Hooray for me! I'm great! A lot of other people would give up. I don't allow negative thoughts. They are not permitted.

- Flying is safer than driving, you know.
- I will exercise more than usual prior to flying; it gets all the brain endorphins going in the right direction and it helps me to relax. I'll exercise when I get home, too.
- I will welcome delays. This will be a challenge to me. I want them so I can get used to them. They will help me overcome my fears. I look forward to them. I can test myself and go to new ground. This is important. I have experienced weather delays and mechanical delays successfully. I'm great and I'm proud.
- Remember, I am flying to overcome my fears. I will treat this as an assignment. I will succeed in my assignment. I can do this. I am strong. You bet I am. Even when I don't feel like it, I show I can do it. I acknowledge my fears and move on.
- I have developed the confidence to cope with panic attacks, too—very successfully. I can do it on a train, in a car, in the desert. I can cope easily with flying and I look forward to it. I've been in training for three years to make this comeback. Good for me!
- When I return from my flight, I'll get a massage or buy myself a new dress, or go to a gymnastics meet for a reward.
- By flying, I get to enhance my confidence, see my friends and family, see the most spectacular views in the world, eat healthy food, exercise, ski, ride horses, and hike all over the world.
- Since the earthquake, I've had to rebuild my belief system, which includes flying. I can trust in flying, and I will trust in flying. I must trust in flying. Every day we put our trust in people and people put their trust in me. It all must work.
- There is no danger in turbulence. It is just part of flying.

- If oxygen masks drop, this is acceptable. Breathe calmly and easily. I am okay and I am fine. The first time might be scary, but the crew has been taught this, and we are fine. This is just preventative.
- I must remember that if strange thoughts pop into my head, I have a faulty information system that is being replaced by education. I am educating myself and I am fine. I replace all faulty thoughts with rational thinking. I am a rational thinker. I will not allow negative images in my brain or in my thought patterns.
- And another thing, shallow breathing is not lack of oxygen but rather an abundance of carbon dioxide. I'm just fine and breathing easily. I rarely have these events anymore, and if I do, I am most adept at handling them. Oh boy, have I had practice.
- I realize my hearing improves when I fly. It is normal, and I am happy to identify noises and be alert. This is part of anxiety and it comes and goes, and I am proud of this ability. I do not allow negative thoughts into my brain. *No!*
- I can fly. I do not allow any silly, negative thoughts into my thinking pattern. I am safe.

Within one year, I was able to begin flying all over the country again, and since then I've gone back to traveling the globe. This experience taught me something, though. For most of my life, when things got difficult for me, I would eat. This time something difficult happened, and I didn't eat. In my own self-analysis, I was able to understand that my brain had the capacity to tell myself to eat or not eat. Here was one experience in my life where I could prove to myself that I didn't *have* to eat to survive. Though I learned this concept intellectually, it could not stave off future eating compulsions. All these years later, I am finally at peace knowing that for some of us, food can be an addictive substance the same way alcohol or drugs can keep you on a quest for more and more and more. In my case, it wasn't just my fears, failures, or feelings. I was facing a true food addiction.

Face Your Lack of Self-Esteem

By day I'm a reality star on the show *Hoarders*®—I wear shorts, tennis shoes, steel-toed boots, hazmat suits, masks, gloves, protective eyewear, respirators, rain gear, and bug spray. By night I'm a vixen (oh, come on—so I wish)! At 200-plus pounds, it didn't matter whether I was in a guerilla costume or a ball gown; I could not ease into my inner beauty. I couldn't get inside, around, or through my physical being—that is, the pounds—to see or understand that there was some femininity in me to be expressed. That was my external self (my body), and it was a reality, and I suffered. But even worse was the monologue I had in my head.

Oh dear, there were too many moments when I just didn't feel smart enough, good enough, or pretty enough. Put on the blindfolds and plug the ears—what I did in my mind is not fit for consumption. If I had known the secret to assembling self-esteem, I certainly would have used it sooner. I had way too many conversations about myself with myself, and really, who cared? It wasn't until I joined a 12-step program that I got clear on how to obtain self-esteem.

It was simple: stop trying to build myself up and start building up others. I was so busy collecting line items for my résumé to impress you, I was forgetting to ask *about* you. That selfishness kept life pretty shallow for me and didn't do much to boost my self-esteem. It seemed like the more I accomplished, the less satisfaction I felt.

I took on the suggestions about really helping to build up others' sense of self-worth, and in doing so, my own self-esteem solidified. The more I praised and complimented others, the better I felt about myself. Okay, why didn't I know about *this* secret system? Jeepers! Working on *Hoarders*® was a perfect forum in which to demonstrate the building up of others. Being in touch with other like-minded

individuals who were concerned about their weight gain was also a
key to success.

I reached out to the members of my program and started sharing, comparing, and changing. While drivers on the road were still
flipping me off because I was driving too slow, or cashiers were still
in bad moods while they were ringing up my groceries, or the TSA
workers at the airport refused to smile at me when I came through
their security lane, I remained cool, confident, and compassionate.
Their attitudes were the same—but I was finally changing.

About fifty pounds down on the scale, I was offered two tickets to
attend the Grammys. This would be my very first Red Carpet event
as a reality star (and not a well-known one at that). Without any of
the ping-pong-ball conversations bouncing around in my head, I
said, "Yes." First, there was no panic about what to wear; I was
becoming thin again, and all those anxious moments were gone.

Next, I had maintained a super relationship with my ex-boyfriend,
and I asked him to join me. Finally, rather than comparing myself
to the gorgeous runway models and celebrities walking alongside
me on the Red Carpet, I embraced my newly developed self-esteem,

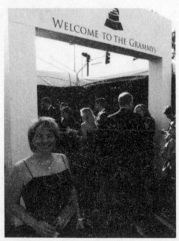

said yes to the sequin dress, and
had my chariot drop me at the edge
of the carpet. Twittering every ten
minutes, I rubbed elbows with the
rich, the famous, and the very tal-
ented. I really wasn't anyone special
that night—it was the Grammys.
I was there to celebrate others'
accomplishments, and boy, did it
feel great!

*Walking the Red Carpet at the
Grammys: Self-esteem in my purse!*

Current Research on Self-Esteem

Many of us wonder whether we do or do not have self-esteem issues. How do you know? Perhaps a good self-esteem test like the Rosenberg Self-Esteem Scale (RSES), developed by sociologist Dr. Morris Rosenberg, can guide you. It is straight to the point and widely used in countries throughout the world. The RSES captures your thoughts by gauging whether you strongly agree or disagree with the statements given.

On the RSES scale, five of the items have positively worded statements and five have negatively worded ones. Take a few minutes to see how you rank.

Rosenberg Self-Esteem Scale

3	2	1	0
strongly agree	agree	disagree	strongly disagree

1. I feel that I am a person of worth, at least on an equal plane with others.
2. I feel that I have a number of good qualities.
3. All in all, I am inclined to feel that I am a failure. (R)
4. I am able to do things as well as most people.
5. I feel I do not have much to be proud of. (R)
6. I take a positive attitude toward myself.
7. On the whole, I am satisfied with myself.
8. I wish I could have more respect for myself. (R)
9. I certainly feel useless at times. (R)
10. At times I think that I am no good at all. (R)

For the items marked with an (R), reverse the scoring (0 = 3, 1 = 2, 2 = 1, 3 = 0). For those items without an (R) next to them, simply add the score. Then, add the scores together. Typical scores on the Rosenberg Scale are around 22, with most people scoring between 15 and 25. *Source:* Copyright and permission granted. Rosenberg, Morris. 1989. "Society and the Adolescent Self-image." Revised edition, Middleton, CT: Wesleyan University Press.

This is one of several scales used to measure self-esteem. If you truly feel you may have problems, seeing a therapist may reveal vulnerabilities that you have stuffed down for way too long. Don't wait for the bottom to fall out. You're much more valuable than the badge of self-neglect.

How Low Self-Esteem Ties Back to Food and Gaining Weight

Low self-esteem relates to food and potential weight gain (or other addictive behaviors), which manifests itself in feeling bad about yourself and possible self-destruction. The perfect companion called "food" loves to feed into your negative thought patterns and feelings of worthlessness. Try letting this partner go, and it will kick and scream to get back into your life like an obsessed spouse who doesn't want to agree to a divorce. Feeling good means reaching out to friends and family who care, and not reaching out to the seductive food, which means guaranteed pounds on the body.

Organizing Tips for Gaining Self-Esteem

My friend Jeanette and her husband, Kevin, are givers—time, money, ideas, support, and solutions. Not only do they give, but they give before they're asked. I have no idea how these two learned all of these life lessons. I'm just grateful they are in my life to teach me. In times of my own lack of self-esteem, Jeanette was always around to remind me of my accomplishments and ask me probing questions that would unlock my confidence again. She also gently reminded me that charitable "doings," as she calls them, feed our inner self, our self-esteem. She knows what it's like to feel great about herself because she gives to others.

It's true: I do belong to or sit on the board for several philanthropic groups, such as Aid Still Required (helping others when natural disaster hits), or the Venice Family Clinic (serving the needs of the uninsured), or many individuals in the world who cannot afford to clear out their hoarded-out homes (we provide pro bono services). Yes, like everything else, if your self-esteem is lacking, it's time to take action and fill the void.

Here are some suggestions to consider:

- What made you smile or laugh this past week?
- What did you feel good about this past week?
- What kinds of things make you feel most relaxed or exhilarated?
- Is there something in particular you feel passionately about?
- How can you nurture yourself today?

Here are some actions to consider:

- Write down some of your favorite places to visit or things you like to do that make you feel good about yourself. Put the ideas in a fishbowl, and whenever you need a boost, pull out an idea.
- Music can feed your soul. Dig out some of your favorite CDs or click on your top iTunes selections and play the songs—loudly!
- Sign up for a class or seminar to learn a new skill or enhance a current talent.
- Read a book about the life of a strong woman, man, or leader.
- Tell someone why you are special today.
- Ask someone else why he or she is special.
- Ask yourself why you are here on this earth and write down the positive answers in your journal.
- Write a thank-you note to someone who encourages you or inspires you.
- Make a list of twelve of your strengths.

Just Not Smart Enough, You See

I mentioned Landmark Education earlier (known to many as the Landmark Forum). My friend Evan Green introduced me to it, and it was here where I moved from being a victim to being bold. I learned that for most of my life I had been suffering from some silly fifth-grade thinking that "I'm not smart enough." *Ridiculous realization*, I thought at the time. Well, now, wait a minute. . . . I remember sitting in a science class as a ten-year-old. My science teacher kept asking questions, and over and over I watched everyone's hands go up to answer his question. Mine did not. I was embarrassed. He would ask more questions, and hands flew up. I just didn't understand the material; it didn't make sense to me.

I was too young to know that I could have just said, "Mr. Scott, I don't understand." Instead, I sat in fear of being stupid, and eventually he called on me. The answers still didn't come. Despite his coaching and the whispers from surrounding classmates, I could not come up with the answer. I spent an adult lifetime hiding out in fear of not being "smart enough." During my training at Landmark Education, I was able to completely decide that I *was* smart enough and I could always ask clarifying questions. The handcuffs were off and I finally had full use of my hands (and my brain).

Well, if I could go from being stupid to being smart in an instant, couldn't I go from being a victim of divorce and deceit to a bold businesswoman? Ah, yeah! Guess who picked up the phone and called the *Dr. Phil* show? The word was out that Dr. Phil's producers were looking for a time management specialist, and I decided it was me (heck, I had just started writing a book on the subject, why not?). I called producers at the studio and learned that, in fact, they were doing a show about a man whose personal style was stuck in the 1960s. He had hair down to his bum, was traveling too much on business, and he never had enough time for his wife. Their marriage was on the brink. Could I help? Yes. Did I have a book? Yes. Er, um, sort of. It was written, but, well, uh, not published. I had never published a book before! Zoiks, Batman, what to do?

Luckily, I had just gone into partnership with my then-clients, now business partners, Debby, Ken, and Lynn. If I were ever to learn what it was like to be in a trusting relationship, it would be with these three individuals. Having come from a traumatic past with lies and deception, I was able to forge a business partnership and a supporting friendship that would change my life. I think that's where I learned how valuable relationships can be in terms of healthy living. It's the reason I've written a separate chapter about it in this book.

You see, Debby, Ken, and Lynn were also taking their life experiences and turning them into service for others. Debby and Ken had *both* of their fathers living with them in their home and together, with Lynn as our lead writer, had written other books about our aging parents (*The Senior Organizer*), interviewing our parents to collect and store their valuable life stories (*Cherished Memories*), and documentaries about keeping our parents safe (*Saving Our Parents*).

These products were born out of near tragedy when Debby and Ken had to rescue Ken's father from a crooked caregiver. Just as most of us do when our parents age, we arrange for a caregiver to come in and stay with them, especially if we are working. What Ken soon found out was that this caregiver was poisoning his father, money was being siphoned out of his father's bank account, and a marriage was being planned so the caregiver could become the recipient of the estate when Ken's father passed away. They, too, had been duped and had to learn to trust, and together we formed a very strong partnership. Naturally, we discussed everything, including how we could get this time management book (*Time Efficiency Makeover*) published by the time I appeared on the *Dr. Phil* show. Did someone say bold?

A Little Chicken Soup for My Soul

Why, I had just finished reading Jack Canfield's book *The Success Principles* and page 139 parked itself in my mind. The title of the chapter is, "ASK! ASK! ASK!" So I did. I called Jack Canfield's office—you know, the co-creator of the wildly popular *Chicken Soup for the Soul* series (oh, no, not again . . . what is it with my picking up the phone and just calling very important people like they are my friend next door?). Well, it was his idea. I told him when he, himself, Jack Canfield, the guy on the front of the book, picked up the phone! It was after 6:00 PM. I had talked myself into being bold yet again, and I dialed the number, ready to leave a really fast message and get the heck off the phone. Except *he* answered! Ah, yeah, Jack Canfield.

So I chanted *his* success principles quickly in my mind:

- Ask as if you expect to get it.
- Assume you can.
- Ask someone who can give it to you.
- Be clear and specific.

Amused, Jack listened to my story about getting a spot on the *Dr. Phil* show and having a book written—but that it was still unpublished. I needed to have a published book to give to the audience in about two months when the *Dr. Phil* taping would take place. Jack introduced me to his company president, Patty, and she opened the doors to my finding a publisher—Health Communications Inc. (HCI)—the very publishers of this book today.

Debby, Lynn, and I went on to coauthor, with Jack Canfield and Mark Victor Hansen, one of our bestselling books at the time—*Life Lessons for Busy Moms: 7 Essential Ingredients to Organize and Balance Your World*. I could never have imagined that my life could be as successful as it was becoming. There were just two areas of life left to learn about: men and finally claiming my own "right-size" body.

Face Your Feelings

Sharma's office was not easy to get to. Oh, let's face it, anywhere in Los Angeles is a difficult commute. Once settled in her dimly lit office with a choice of couches and chairs, plenty of tissues, and oddly no clock, I would start telling Sharma what had happened the week prior. I would list the upsets and the wrongdoings, the mishandlings and the confrontations, and somewhere in each conversation, my therapist would ask me two things: (1) How do you feel about that? and (2) What can you do to make yourself feel better? You know—nurture yourself.

Let me tell you one thing. I love Sharma. Hands down the best therapist I've ever had, but couldn't she change up the questions a little bit? I remember telling Sharma how an ex-boyfriend, Dale, jumped off my balcony and broke his ankle. I gave her the details, I presented the facts, I delivered the story—and then came the question, "Dorothy, how did you feel about that?"

"Jumpin' Jehoshaphats, I don't know, Sharma," I clipped. I would shift positions and stare back at her as though she were the one who was slightly off. The truth is that I had no feelings. I recited to her how *others* felt about that situation.

I recounted the events that logically led up to this bizarre balcony jump, and I could factually explain what I thought I should do next, but how I *felt* about it? Nah. I've got nothing. Empty vessel. No feelings. I needed to fill it (the vessel—I mean, my stomach) instead of *feel* it (you know, the feelings). I could, however, always answer Sharma's second question about what I could do to make myself feel better. I was open and willing: manicure, walk on the beach, see a new movie, go pet some horses at the ranch in the canyon. Secretly, though, I knew what I really would do—hit the bakery on Saturday morning and fill the pink box with twelve perfectly circular, frosting-laden goodies. Indeed, I *filled* the empty vessel, because I sure wasn't feelin' it.

Looking back on my early work with Sharma, I realize that she had to ask those two questions repeatedly because she was training me to manage my own feelings. I would go to her every week for years because I didn't know how to do it for myself. Now, when a situation arises, I hear Sharma's voice and I can ask myself those questions. I'm such a slow learner sometimes. But I got it, Sharma, I got it.

Sharma had also given me several books over the course of our work together. I remember one book titled *Food for the Soul*, which included a four-sentence checklist to review feelings:

1. Anger is the feeling I get when I don't get my way today.
2. Resentment is the feeling I get when I think about having not gotten my way yesterday.
3. Fear is the feeling I get when I worry that I won't get my way tomorrow.
4. Depression is the feeling I get when I sit around wondering why I never get my way.

I believe that any one of these emotions is brought on by a slow buildup of even the smallest of upsets that occur in our lives. In fact, I now notice that when you allow one small upset into your life, it's like a magnet—lots of upsets start following. Just like when you open a bag of chips: you just allow one into your mouth and *boom*! Before you know it, the whole bag is gone! They just magically flow from the bag into your mouth. Have you ever experienced this? So it is with small upsets.

Example: A cashier is amazingly rude to you at the store—a small upset. You think about it on your way to the car, you get distracted, you replay the conversation, and you begin having an emotional obsession. While putting the bags in the trunk, you clunk your head, still thinking about the nasty cashier. Your head hurts from the clunk and your brain hurts from the conversation about the cashier over the junk in your trunk.

Distracted, you drive and miss your turn, and you have to make a separate U-turn and come back around. Now, a driving jerk won't let you in (small upset), you're stuck in traffic going the other direction (small upset), you are now late for your appointment (small upset), you are rather nasty to others at your next appointment (small upset)—can you see the domino effect? Now, you could go this route or simply dismiss the conversation from the cashier at the get-go. You could thank her, wish her a pleasant day, and say to yourself every time the thought of that nasty cashier comes up, *I don't care to think about that right now. I'm busy being happy and content!*

Upsets and the feelings caused from those upsets, or any other precious, happy, or delicate moments, come up each and every day. We can certainly ask ourselves Sharma's two therapy session questions, and we can also learn a little something from another prominent doctor of emotions, Charlene Miller.

Current Research on Feelings

My friend and colleague Dr. Charlene Underhill Miller is a licensed marriage, family, and child therapist in California who provides psychotherapy to individuals, couples, and families and treats a wide range of issues such as self-sabotage, parenting challenges, eating disorders, hoarding, and addictions. She shares about her clients' feelings and their relationship to food.

> Jill had been sexually abused by her stepfather from the age of six until she told this haunting secret at the age of fourteen. Shipped off to a girls' home, she never received effective therapy and never talked about it. As a young mother of three, Jill arrived at my office because she wanted to understand her feelings of depression, anxiety, and her difficulty of bonding to her children the way she thought a mother should. Jill was despondent and had gained enough weight over the years that she had no noticeable shape, felt sexually unattractive, and had put literal physical distance between her body and the threat of another man's abuse.
>
> Separately, Ida had grown up in an emotionally distant and cruel family. Her mother criticized and mocked her for eating too much as

a child. Ida began to hoard her food and began what became a lifetime of secret bingeing. When life felt stressful or when she felt lonely, Ida found comfort in the food she had hoarded for herself. She loved food like she might love a person. Ida not only became addicted to food but became addicted to acquiring the food; she knew every fast-food restaurant on her way home from work, and plotting her way, she stopped at no less than five. Ida knew she needed to handle her loneliness and stress much differently. By the time she came to therapy, she was obese, depressed, and financially strapped.

Gloria learned her compulsive eating patterns from her mother. She watched her mother talk to food like it was a lover and at other times like it was the enemy. Food was part of every celebration and sorrow. Food was her mother's way of soothing Gloria's hurt feelings. Gloria's mother never really talked about feelings; she just stuffed them. So, too, did Gloria.

Being soothed with food is perhaps our earliest experience. Mother's milk is provided soon after we are born. We are comforted and held. We are adored and nurtured. And as time goes on, this hopefully translates to a wonderful and complex relationship with our parents, who provide nurture in a variety of ways. However, our unhealthy relationship with food can often begin very early in our childhood, and we often unconsciously replicate the patterns of our parents and their parents. Sometimes we are rewarded with food and sometimes food is withheld from us as punishment. An unhealthy relationship with food begins, and it is difficult to see food as just f-o-o-d.

Parents either don't or don't know how to model healthy communication about painful issues. Many families ignore painful life experiences. Deaths and divorces often get pushed under the rug. Financial difficulties get whispered about. Children and their feelings are often ignored and minimized. When they see their parents having emotional struggles, children often experience anxiety and depression. For many this is the time that dysfunctional eating begins.

Gloria found herself hoarding her favorite candy, storing it under her bed in preparation for her parents' fights. Ida remembers sitting on her back porch consuming an entire pan of lasagna, relishing in the warm and connected feelings she experienced as she swallowed the melted cheese. And Jill remembers eating a whole chocolate cake one day after her stepfather molested her. It was her way of connecting to her mother, a mother who never addressed her daughter's abuse and pretended not to notice that it was going on. Each of these women ended up choosing spouses who replicated the pain and abuse they experienced from their primary parents. Sometimes we unconsciously gravitate to relational experiences and ways of coping that are most familiar—even when those ways are destructive.

As with many addictions, the tendency to abuse food happens when one is hungry, angry, lonely, or tired. Those familiar with 12-step philosophy use the acronym HALT. We are likely to eat more than we need when we are too hungry. We eat ravenously, like we will never get food again. And rather than expressing our angry feelings in a constructive and appropriate way, we stuff our anger by bingeing on food until our anger subsides and depression begins. And sometimes food becomes our "lover" when we are most lonely. Standing in front of a refrigerator or pantry eating through the night may be the quickest remedy for rejection. And when we are the most tired, we are often the most vulnerable to disordered eating. We have exhausted ourselves helping others all day; we haven't taken very good care of ourselves, and so our eating is our "reward"; it's just a dysfunctional reward.

Paying attention to our emotions helps us understand our triggers for disordered eating. Facing and understanding these feelings often is most helpful in the company of a good friend, a group, and often an understanding therapist. Facing one's lifetime of feelings, issues, pain, and family difficulties takes courage and patience. This cannot be done alone. When one has consulted friends or support groups and still feels burdened by disordered eating, perhaps it is time to consult a therapist in order to face the feelings that have led to the eating issues. Here are some helpful things to keep in mind when deciding to seek professional help.

- Consult your support network (physician, religious or spiritual mentor, friends) for a good referral to a licensed therapist who understands issues that contribute to disordered eating.
- Consult with a few of these therapists to see who might be a good therapeutic fit for you. Good therapeutic fit takes into account the professional experience of the therapist, the fee, the location, and your own personal comfort level with that therapist.
- Understand that addressing a lifetime of issues that has led to a lifetime of stuffing feelings takes time. Most good relationships, including therapeutic relationships, take time to develop. People who have suffered tremendous breaches of trust throughout their lifetime may have some difficulty establishing a therapeutic relationship.
- Your therapist should help you understand your family of origin and how early attachments with your mother and father were made. Was food a primary way of coping for your family? Did they communicate directly or indirectly (or not at all) about family issues, feelings, difficulties, pain, and loss? Was food a coping tool for terrible breaches of trust?
- Your therapist should help you understand how you have transferred much of your childhood pain onto your current relationships and how difficult relationships contribute to your disordered eating and bingeing.
- Your therapist should help you become more conscious about your feelings and your relationships where you begin to make intentional and conscious shifts in how you cope.

- Your therapist should help you understand that feelings are okay and necessary and that there are healthy ways of communicating that you are hurt, angry, lonely, or tired.
- Your therapist should help you with healthy coping tools and resources like books, groups, journals, letters, and family therapy, which can allow you to live a healthy and functional life.

When Jill, Ida, and Gloria entered therapy, they began having some important insights about their eating. They each began to understand the themes behind their eating—how food had become a way of coping from significant pain, how food had become a way to push down their feelings, and how food had become a way to express their feelings. In telling their painful histories in a safe and empathetic environment, they each began to understand how food had never been an adequate coping mechanism, but had been a way they perpetuated their life pain by abusing themselves. Self-sabotage is a common way of taking back the control in one's life; it just isn't a productive way.

Jill, Ida, and Gloria made commitments to replace their disordered eating with healthier ways of taking care of themselves. They learned how to create healthy relational boundaries, consciously chose healthier love relationships and friendships, and continue to pursue healthy ways of communicating their feelings, needs, wants, and desires. They are committed to a lifetime of facing their feelings rather than stuffing their faces.

Whether you think you can or whether you think you can't, you're right.

—*Henry Ford*

Since its inception, the Delphi Center for Organization's dedicated staff member Gilliam Drake has always reached for excellence in both business and friendship. Her vision of what it takes to face the emotional leads us to create positive gifts and high energy. Based on her research from the Mayo Clinic website, Gillian gives several examples of problem areas, followed by practical suggestions on how to sweep away negative feelings.

The power of positive thought: Is it really all in your head? Do you let negative self-talk and beliefs about your abilities, intellect, or education adversely affect your possibilities for achievements and success? If your heart's in the right place, anything is possible. You can achieve your goals through positive thought—you hear it all the time—but there's a logical reason that it works. And many gurus of our day believe that expressing your gratitude to others, in a journal, to an Ultimate Power, or to the universe can make a difference in how much you have to be grateful for. So is it really all in your head, or do you have to put more of your heart into it?

When changing our behavior or trying to achieve any goal—whether eating and weight loss, decluttering and better organization, growing our businesses, or pursuing a goal or life dream—some positive psychology might help. Current positive psychological practices are an outgrowth of the 1968 research by Robert Rosenthal, a Harvard University professor, and Leonore Jacobson, an elementary school principal who reported what was called the Pygmalion effect, a phenomenon in which students often performed to the level of expectation placed upon them.[1] It is believed that the Pygmalion effect is a form of self-fulfilling prophecy, in that we internalize projected expectations—whether our own or others'—and perform to them, whether negatively or positively.

James Rhem, executive editor for the online National Teaching and Learning Forum, says, "When teachers expect students to do well and show intellectual growth, they do; when teachers do not have such expectations, performance and growth are not so encouraged and may in fact be discouraged in a variety of ways. How we believe the world is and what we honestly think it can become have powerful effects on how things will turn out."

Many of us eat emotionally in response to stress, and many of us create a good deal of stress for ourselves with "stories" about our stuff—how things won't turn out right, how we won't perform well, or that we just don't have enough skills to accomplish our goals. When we do this, according to the Pygmalion effect, we are doubly sabotaging our own possibilities for achievement and success: causing additional stress that can drive us to continue our overeating and discourage ourselves with negative self-talk.

Gillian reminded me that it's important to insert some positive vibrations into your home and life. Check in with yourself for any old stories—the "I can't do this" kind of self-talk, self-criticism or negativity, perceived rejection by others, or old arguments or attitudes that you may be hanging on to. Give yourself permission to purge and replace or review.

- Replace "can't" with "won't," and then ask yourself why you won't.
- Replace self-criticism with a positive affirmation about yourself.
- Replace perceived rejection by another with a more probable explanation—they were simply preoccupied with their own life or troubles.

Choosing to swap some negative habits for some positive ones means getting rid of things that have not produced good results in your life and identifying things that no longer work for you. It means changing and updating the way you do things, which will free up some space in your life for new and exciting opportunities and challenges. Cleaning up your life needs a dedicated effort, and if you slide one day, it means picking up the ball the next—without beating yourself up! Having a positive attitude is just that: it's a conscious choice. But something interesting happens when you do: you change the way other people perceive you, and—believe it or not—the way you feel about yourself and the way you act.

Here are some ideas to get you started:

- Scrub up your attitude. Showing kindness and love toward others changes the way others treat you. Open friendships require forgiveness, understanding, and thoughtfulness. Going the extra mile for someone shows you care, but remember, friendships should be reciprocal—no one wants to be a doormat. Petty misunderstandings and frazzled impatience can pile up; a diet of gossipy chitchat, rumor spreading, and lies will weigh you down. Take out the trash and own up to your mistakes; a simple apology can put the sparkle back into any friendship.

- Polish up your rocking chair and meditate on the things that are important in your life. Do you live in the moment? "Woulda, Coulda, Shoulda" is such a sad song! Delay and procrastination makes you late, frustrated, or a failure. You'll find yourself missing deadlines, rushing, stressed, or angry and disappointed. So be present and act now, not later. Only make realistic to-do lists, and always add one enjoyable thing a day to your list—even if it's only reading the news with a cup of coffee!

- Dirty, "energy-draining" emotions—being jealous, self-doubting, quick or smoldering anger—clean them up! Negative thoughts and feelings are toxic; they add nothing beneficial to your life and are simply not worth hanging on to. Think of them as dirty laundry. You can leave it in the laundry basket for only so long before it starts to stink. You have to wash your favorite T-shirt so that you can enjoy wearing it again! Otherwise it's just going to stay smelly! We all love the way fabric softener makes our clothes smell. Think of positive thoughts as fabric softener for your mind.

- Dust off your gratitude! Studies show that positively focusing on all the things you appreciate and are grateful for in your life actually changes your perspective. You will find that the more things you appreciate, the more things you will attract into your life to appreciate. And being grateful naturally stops your negative thoughts—you will be happier!

- Clean the windows of your mind to let in the light—new ideas and fresh perspectives. Clean windows allow us to see things outside more clearly and also shed light within. Change doesn't happen overnight, but when you can see more clearly, it's easier to take action to change. By gradually practicing some positive life-cleaning chores, you can create new habits, be the person you truly want to be, and create the life you truly want.

Face Your Toxic Relationships

It's Raining Men

Tracy is addicted to men. Instead of alcohol, she seeks another guy, and another guy, and another guy—one after the next. Suffering from a "please love me, but stay away" syndrome, Tracy shops for clothes, cosmetics, wigs, hair accessories, and beauty supplies to look good and attract men. Her fear of being alone is so great that she has filled her home with so much stuff from thrift stores and discount houses that it repels the very men she attracts. The men who do show a lingering interest and who are willing to overlook Tracy's hoard are themselves a bit unstable, bringing further toxicity into her home. Her addiction to men motivates her to look pulled together, but her appearance is the disguise that covers up her hoarded-out living conditions. Her home is so full of purchases and secret deals (items with sale price tags still in the bag from the stores), even her children have fled the home to live with other family members. Lonely and now without family, Tracy regularly summons up her standby routine: shopping. She goes out to buy more flashy clothing, a new curling iron, and more anti-wrinkle cream, and is off to meet the next knight in shining armor—who always winds up riding off in the other direction. The cycle never ends.

Food was likely the first of my toxic relationships. But wait a second, you say. Aren't relationships supposed to be with people? Yessss. The red flag was waving! Danger was all around me. That's why I'm telling you this. I treated food like my companion, my friend, my turn-to-in-any-crisis confidante. Folks, I am here to tell you that if you maintain a toxic relationship with someone or something, the need for self-care is paramount. If there was any relationship on the planet that needed to be nurtured, it was the one I had with myself.

You see, I was a woman of extremes. I was an either-or kind of gal. One or the other, hot or cold. I had very little consistency in my life, and only in therapy did I learn the extraordinary value of structure and consistency for myself.

Let me demonstrate what life used to be like for me:

I'm One Way . . .	Or	The Other
I was busier than ever	or	I was excruciatingly bored.
I was careless	or	I was meticulous.
I was eating recklessly	or	I was eating strictly.
I was embarrassed and overweight	or	I was sassy and skinny.
I drove a broken-down van that I started with a screwdriver	or	I drove a snappy classic Jaguar like Lady Diana.
My bedroom was in total upheaval and disarray	or	My bedroom was immaculate and pristine.
My clothes were schlumpy	or	My clothes were impeccable.
My life was traumatic	or	My life was charmed.

Got the picture? My life was inconsistent and very difficult to keep straight, for me and everyone around me. Is Dorothy dieting or should we have some treats for when she visits? Should we dress up for Dorothy's dinner party or do you think she's in her "I don't care" mode? How confusing! I swear, I could not figure out from one week to the next how I would be able to bounce back from my latest personal disaster. All wound up, I would sit in heavy, slow-moving Los Angeles traffic to get to Sharma's office for my weekly therapy sessions. Yes, she gave me real-time tools; yes, I was able to vent and regroup. No matter what, Sharma reminded me of that one thing that was always last on my list—taking care of me.

That's why I think that addressing relationships is so important in terms of losing weight and setting your life straight. Speaking of relationships and looking back on my days of working with Sharma, I brought everyone in my life with me to my therapy sessions— all of my family members, my ex-husband, and boyfriends. *They* all needed the help, so I thought. In my crazy thinking, I always thought it was the *other* person who needed the help! It was so easy for me to see in others what they needed to work on, fix, or change, so I took them to Sharma. To be fair, I needed to learn that a person like me who creates a toxic relationship with food is likely to seek other toxic relationships, too, and that's exactly what I did in terms of picking relationships as a young adult. While this did not happen to me in business, I unknowingly sought out toxic intimate relationships and wound up dragging all of my loved ones into the world of counseling, therapy, self-reflection, and transformation.

I suppose I felt like I was growing and learning, and I was worried that perhaps they were not. But honestly, I don't think I knew how to express my own needs to the important people around me. With my ex-husband or boyfriends, I wasn't even able to decipher whether the relationships were healthy for me or not. My "man selection" button was not in proper working order, and for everyone else in my life,

I didn't want to cause upset by stating my needs. So off we went to Sharma, where I found myself able to communicate in a safe zone.

Men in Trees

Let's talk about the men thing for a moment, shall we? After my divorce, and despite being on my way to hard-fought success in business, I got involved with another guy a bit too much like my ex-husband. His name was Dale, but he was really Bob. Huh? What I mean to say is I picked the same kind of guy all over again. Why, why, why?

I guess it was because I didn't have the capacity or know-how to love and take care of myself. I didn't really have a great diet, I worked unusually long hours, I wasn't getting enough sleep, I didn't schedule necessary doctors' appointments, and I had very little recreation. Couldn't I just get the love and care I needed from a guy? No, Dorothy, the Wizard of Oz is not accepting requests today. I just couldn't figure it out, and it's why I am presenting specific chapters in this book to you about health, sleep, and creating your goals and dreams.

I could tell from the get-go of my relationship with Dale that it wasn't really right for me, because I began overeating from the very start. First, I thought it was just because we were dining out at exclusive restaurants, sharing bottles of wine, and strolling for fine chocolates before turning in for the evening. Dale had lots of money to spend, and he wanted to spend it on me. I was wrapped up in the world of fantasy and delusion. Just when I was at the peak of my early popularity and success, I found myself ignoring my responsibilities. Staying up all night, dining, and dancing disrupted my sleep, and I had considered myself a morning person! Suddenly I wasn't. I couldn't get up in the morning like I used to, I nixed any exercise, and I found myself skipping breakfast—and sometimes skipping work. Dale convinced me that he would take care of me, something I had not experienced in my adult lifetime, as I never really could count on Bob. The idea of being taken care of was enchanting.

Silly as it may seem, at forty-two, I remember Dale taking me to Disneyland for the first time in my life. We got preferred parking, we got special VIP passes, we jumped to the head of every line, rode every ride, got sugar treats in every confectionary shop, and dined in the upscale restaurants. It was Christmastime at Disneyland and the carolers were singing, the night parade was glowing, the fireworks were busting out overhead, and Dale took me into a store and said, "Dorothy, you can have anything you want in this store. Just pick it out and I'll buy it for you."

Immediately, I relived the happiest moments of my childhood, hand in hand with my dad, with him telling me I could pick out any doughnut in the bakery. It was weird, and from that moment on, whether it made sense or not, I viewed Dale as the guy who could take care of me for the rest of my life. Except he couldn't. Dale had other women who were just as important to him, and he made the same promises to the others as he did to me.

I've learned that if I can't figure myself out, I have no business being in a relationship. Indeed, I had not figured myself out; therefore, I had trouble getting myself out of another relationship that was not healthy for me. Over a year into my relationship with Dale, my intuition proved to be correct. Obvious evidence of infidelity, which I could not avoid, presented itself to me (okay, I looked at Dale's phone bill, which indicated that he was calling someone every night before bed). Dale had been dating another woman seriously, and in addition to asking for my hand in marriage, he had proposed to her as well. Nice lady. I talked to her. We compared notes. Where exactly is my made-for-TV movie script for the Lifetime channel, folks? The good news is that with Bob it took me sixteen years to get out of the relationship—actually it was done for me—and it took me less than two years to get out of this one. I was improving but still had more work to do.

One evening I pressed Dale on the subject of having an affair, and he didn't like it at all. I could see his temperature gauge rising, and I recall telling him that he needed to get out of my life now and for good. He didn't want to. Dale told me he wasn't leaving! After what seemed like hours of harassment and fights, I called the police to come and remove him from my third-floor apartment.

Just moments later, the police arrived to collect Dale. I talked to them at my front door and described the situation in detail to them. The police then went into my small two-bedroom apartment to talk to Dale. Dale? Where was Dale? No Dale. Checked in the bathroom behind the shower curtain. No Dale. Under the bed? No Dale. This was preposterous! In the closet? No Dale. Spare room? Nope. Wait. Had the screen been removed from the window? Yes! No, don't tell me Dale jumped? Oh boy, so frightened at the thought of being arrested, Dale jumped from my third-story balcony to a tree branch below and fell to the ground. With a broken ankle, he ran like a criminal to his car. *Is this really my life?* Yes, Dorothy, it is. You've got to figure this thing out. You've got to figure "you" out.

Now, to be fair, I have since talked to Dale all about this. Having just lost his wife prior to our relationship, he admitted he had a lot to come to terms with. Fear of pain and abandonment clouded his judgment. Trust issues dogged me, and I was living each day in a sugar coma. Both of us were coming off very traumatic relationship losses, and we were not a good match at the time. Dale is now a good friend of mine. With apologies and a few laughs exchanged, we agree about how we learned so much back then. Now his supportive friendship is invaluable to me.

Though I had breakthroughs and enlightening experiences with some relationships, not all relationships were healed back then. This was, I believe, because I continued to use food to fill my feelings of emptiness. With so much information and so many experiences, what was it that had me continue to stuff my face? It's easy for me to see now that while I had begun to face my stuff, I still hadn't faced three areas of my life. I had not:

1. Apologized to others or myself for past behaviors or choices, which could relieve me of guilt, anger, and resentment.
2. Joined a community where I felt I belonged. Some people have church or temple, some belong to a motorcycle club; others play bridge or tennis with the same group every month. Me? I was a lone renegade.
3. Developed a spiritual connection. This was completely elusive for me. I had no experience with, or interest in, finding a spiritual connection that was bigger than me. It wasn't on my radar screen to consider, and I certainly didn't know how.

On my own, outside of the counselors and therapists, I needed to find my voice and ask directly to get my needs met. I needed to stop lying to myself about my ex having an affair. I needed to finally be okay with my mom not liking my haircuts or decorating choices. I needed to have tough conversations with friends who were not holding up their end of our friendship and ask that they begin to nurture and take care of themselves, too. For those who owed me money, I asked them to consider paying me back and not letting it go "unsaid" anymore. I also went to those to whom I owed money and reconciled with them.

I used to let everyone dictate how "our" relationship would be designed, and I went along with it. Well, you know what? Once I put down the sugar and flour, I had a lot of new and available time to redesign my relationships, ask for what I wanted or needed, and summon the courage to say bye-bye to the bad seeds in my life and hello to respect and integrity.

Now, when I talk about respect and integrity, I'm talking about respect for myself and integrity to myself. I have finally learned that it all starts with me. In each and every relationship in which I participate, I see that I am responsible—I can no longer blame the other. Looking at my old chaotic relationship patterns has allowed me to create predictable and worthwhile new ones, and I remember the day my understanding of all this shifted.

I began to study personal transformation. Up until the time I began studying transformation, I don't think I ever knew anyone who practiced this kind of self-reflection and development. The concept was new to me, yet the people moving in and among these groups were transforming themselves, and I hoped this would happen for me, too. With other self-growth groupies, I began working through deep questions and answers about myself and looking for areas where I "shared" some responsibility in the breakdown of my relationships with other people in my life. Now, remember, I think I'm joining this group to lose weight, but instead I'm doing an inventory of myself? Really? Yes, Dorothy, really.

To do this, I looked to all the people in my life with whom I held resentments. I asked myself what *they* had done that made *me* feel so resentful. Easy. Ex-husband had an affair. Dearest friend stopped calling me after we had a misunderstanding. A business colleague snubbed me when I'd made a mistake, even after I'd apologized for it. Yes, I could do this step. Further, we were asked to consider "our part" of the deterioration of the relationship. But, surprisingly, this came easily to me, and what I discovered in the nearly fifty-seven situations I listed was that I actually resented myself, not the other people. I was the target of resentment, and I punished myself with food.

- I resented myself for getting involved with my ex-husband, who was twice my age. Even though I was barely legal and had never dated anyone other than my high school sweetheart, I'd been angry with myself for nearly thirty years for being so naive and stupid about this.
- I resented myself for being an accomplice to my diabetic father's

food binges. I never questioned his actions or expressed concern for Dad's health when it came to the food he ate, and I've been living with that guilt for nearly forty years. In fact, I was just a child wanting her dad's love and attention.

- I felt great disappointment in myself when a dear friend of mine suddenly stopped calling and refused to take my calls anymore. I had no idea why she had a change of heart, and like most of the relationships in my life, I took the blame and searched for what I could have done wrong. I have since learned that people who care about me will communicate with me to adjust any miscommunications, even if it's difficult.

Bottom line: For every relationship or situation involving other people that didn't work out, I burdened myself with guilt, anger, resentment, disappointment, and more. Furthermore, I was shocked to learn that I rarely listened to my intuition or my inner voice about making choices in my life.

I asked myself what had happened to that carefree little girl who giggled and ran around nonstop? I closed my eyes and recalled a photo taken of me when I was three years old. I remembered that little pixie and I liked her. I immediately pulled out the bin with all my nostalgic photos and sorted through them until I found that picture. I looked at that sweet little one and knew, like a protective parent, that I would no longer let *that* little girl endure the guilt, anger, resentment, or disappointment anymore. Out came the picture, up went the frame, and I posted that photograph of myself across from my bed to see every morning when I awakened. Is there a young photo of yourself that you might pull out and use as inspiration? I encourage you to find that picture of that sweet child and place it where you can see it daily. You might even ask yourself now and again when making decisions, *Would I let this little pipsqueak hang out with that person, eat that package of cookies right before bed, spend money on that meaningless gadget?*

When I pulled out that picture of myself as an innocent child, I knew I was ready to invest in a healthy relationship with myself, one that I had never known—period. Out of that insight, all of my other relationships experienced a massive shift as well. Setting out to fix all my relationships was not the answer. Changing how I behaved in each of those relationships? Yes—that was the answer.

Current Research on Relationships

Identifying our own flaws in our relationships is a great place to start. There are some real humdinger kinds of words we've said or actions we've taken that we're not proud of. There are also some little picayune details we may be overlooking in terms of our behavior with others. Consider the following situations to see where you fall on the scale of neglectful relationship behavior. Use these scenarios to get to the truth and make a note as to the person who comes to mind when you read each question. This might just be a starting point for you to make some behavior shifts of your own. Go ahead, jot down some names and circle the answers that best apply to you. Just engaging in the questions will bring you closer to facing your stuff, too.

You get home from an evening out and check your messages. Finding several calls from family and friends, you:

1. Phone them all back as soon as you can.
2. Save the messages, settle in, and then call each one back.
3. Save the messages, settle in, and call only the ones you really care about that night and save the rest for another time.
4. Save the messages and then call them back when you get the chance.
5. Forget to call them back.

You are in a romantic relationship that is just not working out for you. You decide to end it, so you:

1. Talk to him or her as soon as you can.
2. Think about it for a week before talking about it.
3. Think about it for a month before talking about it.
4. Try to talk yourself out of ending the relationship.
5. Send an e-mail or leave an answering machine message ending the relationship.
6. Let it drag on and hope he or she breaks up with you.
7. Disappear without contacting the other person.

You arrange to go out with a friend who suggests seeing a movie that you don't want to see, so you:

1. Immediately tell him or her that you don't want to go to that movie.
2. Wait until you get to the theater before telling him or her.
3. Drag your feet so that you miss the movie.
4. Go to the movie in a sour mood.
5. Make an agreement to endure this movie and next time you get to select the movie or activity.

An old friend sent you a birthday gift and now it is a month past your birthday. You:

1. Immediately call and thank your friend for the gift and apologize for not calling sooner.
2. Call in about a week and thank him or her for the gift.
3. Call and pretend you didn't get the gift.
4. Call when you know he or she won't be home so that you're not so embarrassed.
5. Don't call and risk he or she feeling hurt or wondering if you are okay.

When it is your turn to pick up a friend for an outing, you are most often:

1. Right on time.
2. Five to ten minutes late.
3. Ten to fifteen minutes late.
4. Around twenty minutes late.
5. None of the above. Your friends seem to always volunteer to pick you up.

You volunteer to take pictures at your friend's wedding. Do you:

1. Develop the photos immediately?
2. Develop them within the month?
3. Develop them within the year?
4. Not develop them, but always promise you will?
5. Lose the file or photos?

Dr. Barbara De Angelis is an internationally recognized expert on human relations. In her book *Real Moments*, she writes,

An intimate relationship is a sacred opportunity for you to use love as a path for personal and spiritual transformation. It forces you to open where you were closed, to feel where you were numb, to express what was silent, to reach out when you would retreat. It's easy to feel like you are a loving and enlightened person when you are alone, but when you get into a relationship, you come face-to-face with every emotional limitation you possess. Relationships are an instant and continual training ground. They insist that you look in the mirror at yourself; they reveal all the parts of you that are not loving. They show you your dark side. They knock on the door of your heart, demanding that you open the places you've kept locked. And then, every day and night, they give you an opportunity to practice love, to stretch yourself beyond what is comfortable, and to keep doing it better.

Author of the book *Loving What Is*, Byron Katie stresses that it is important to become aware of your stories. Similar to what I talked about earlier in terms of working on Step 4 with my 12-step group, Katie suggests, "Stories appear in our minds hundreds of times a day. Examples are: when someone gets up without a word and walks out of the room; when someone doesn't smile or return a phone call; before you open an important letter, or after you feel an unfamiliar sensation in your chest; when your boss invites you to come into his office, or when your partner talks to you in a certain tone of voice. Stories are the untested, uninvestigated theories that tell us what all these things mean. We don't even realize that they're just theories."

It might be interesting for you to consider how you interpret the actions of other people around you. Generally the actions of others have absolutely nothing to do with us, but we make their actions mean something. Today, as you go through your day, observe yourself when you suddenly feel slighted, ignored, overlooked, or doted upon. How do you interpret others' actions? What if you did not allow yourself to react to others' actions? You may just experience a little extra peace in your day concerning your own relationships.

How Relationships Tie Back to Food and Gaining Weight

It was just a simple question that I would ask my ex-husband: "Did you call the insurance company?" Simple. One question. No long, involved story. Just a question. Please tell me, folks, how a question to my ex-husband about insurance at the end of a workday would cause me to binge on an entire bag of cookies and a quart of milk? I certainly didn't see it then, but I assure you, as I studied how my responsibilities in relationships were not working, I could see it.

Not only was I causing upset between me and my ex, but I was gaining weight by my behavior, too. Here's the answer: I asked only one question, but I asked that same question every night until there was a huge blowup. I also look back and can hear the tone in which I delivered my ever-accusatory question night after night. Somehow, my intention of "being helpful" turned into a nagging wife with an attitude. Let me demonstrate:

1st time:	Did you call the insurance company?	Trying to be helpful, kind voice
2nd time:	Did you call the insurance company?	Reminding, authoritative voice
3rd time:	Did you call the insurance company?	Nagging, aggravating voice
4th time:	Did you call the insurance company?	Harping, accusatory voice
5th time:	Did you call the insurance company?	Controlling, righteous voice

Whether you are the giver or receiver, ultimately this type of escalating and repetitive conversation doesn't feel good. One can also see how we chase others away by nagging, harping, and controlling, *and* we can see how we run away when it's done to us. Either way, this experience causes anxiety, and anxiety often causes us to eat. I asked these kinds of questions nearly every day in my marriage to Bob. I must acknowledge that despite what he may have done to contribute to our relationship breakdown, I owned a lot of it, too. Not wanting to admit any of it back then, my only option was to go to the place where I was understood—food.

Organizing Tips
for Toxic Relationships

I learned so much about relationships from my own mistakes. I also learned much from a book titled *Destructive Relationships* by Dr. Jill Murray, professor of psychology at the American Behavioral Studies Institute and a licensed therapist with a private practice in Laguna Niguel, California. Dr. Murray feels that it is important to establish good boundaries with everyone who comes into contact with you, and she developed a list that features the results of good boundaries. Here are some of her suggestions:

1. Have clear preferences and act upon them.
2. Live actively rather than reactively.
3. Extend yourself to others only when they are appreciative.
4. Trust your intuition.
5. Have your own interests and hobbies that excite you.
6. Know the difference between well-intentioned feedback and manipulation or control.
7. Relate to others only when they show respect for your feelings and opinions.
8. Don't "need" another person to make you feel "complete."
9. Understand that you create your own future, and don't depend on others to do so for you.
10. Don't use denial as a coping mechanism, but see things as they are even if they are painful.

5

CURB THE CHAOS OF LIFE:
Face Your Lack of Sleep and Time (and Overwhelm)

I'm not sure why this is exactly, but I was the type of person who could not hear advice from others. Give advice? Sure thing! Receive it? No way—especially from my mother, my spouse, or friends who were close to me. I was like the secret building on the TV sitcom *Get Smart*, with dungeon doors closing, elevator doors slamming, and grid-iron gates locking. Try to say something to help Dorothy and *boom*! She plugs her ears and sings, "La la la la."

Then some unsuspecting person on the subway or in line at the supermarket or at an industry conference says *the exact same thing* to you (well, me), and *ta-da*! It's like magical information. No kidding? Really? I never knew that. How did you know that, where can I get a book on it, when should I start, do I need to buy anything to make it happen, huh, huh, huh? My hardheaded little self. I could have made my life so much easier if I had only listened, especially to my mom. . . .

Years ago, I remember being in glittery Las Vegas with my then husband and dear friends Rod and Andrea. They had come in from Wisconsin, and we were meeting them in Vegas while they attended another friend's wedding ceremony. Excited to see my sweet friend from the sixth grade, I stayed up late into the night to get all my work done and be clear for my vacation time with Andrea. I worked my regular job as an executive assistant by day and was already running my part-time organizing business on evenings and weekends, which left me *when* to get proper sleep? Uh, never.

In addition to the early "up" in the mornings and the "way-too-late-to-bed" nights, I was running on maybe four hours of sleep, which is probably why I was so sleepy at 2:00 PM and 4:00 PM each day. Identifying my need for sleep wasn't on my radar screen—keeping myself awake was. The most common tool, the *only* tool I used to manage my sleep deprivation, was a little pick-me-up called candy bar, shake, or pastry and coffee—no change there. Perfect! I was falsely stimulated throughout the day until I could no longer take it. There I was in Vegas, walking the Strip, and everyone was in a super-giggly mood, having a blast, and right in front of the dancing waters at Caesar's Palace, where crowds are active and moving about to the music, I declare, "I've gotta lie down immediately. I just can't stay awake."

My ex knew exactly what this meant. I could no longer function, period. I had to sleep, even if only for six to eight minutes. The minute I hit the wall (which was usually every day), my head would pop up like a mole showing his little head through the ground and quickly turning in all directions, searching for a flat surface in which to create my fantasy queen-size bed from home.

Feeling no different from a homeless person looking for a stable night's sleep, I was seeking a quick napping surface. What? Rod, Andrea, Bob, and the others all stopped. "What do you mean you have to sleep?"

I tell them, "It'll be less than ten minutes, I'll be fine—just go ahead and I'll catch up." Still mumbling and already in a sleepy haze, I positioned my backpack on the round, flat surface of the water fountain wall and went directly to sleep. Never mind playing gracious host. Excuse the fact that I left everyone high and dry in favor of my bizarre behavior. I was in a deep state of sleep in just seconds. This happened with all of my friends. Whether having dinner at their home or hiking in Mendocino, I was overcome by a wave of tiredness I could not control. I was positive it was narcolepsy.

Never thinking to review my own sleeping and eating behavior, I marched to my primary physician at UCLA. At the beginning of the appointment, my blood pressure was taken; pulse, too. Naturally, I was weighed, and my doctor would hit me between the eyes with the word "obesity" during most of my visits. She is an excellent doctor and has the highest care in mind for me, but whenever I heard the honest truth come from her mouth to my ears . . . ohhh! Call me the cartoon character Roadrunner, with steam pumping out my ears to the sound of an end-of-the-day work whistle! Not willing to accept that I was overweight and that my own diet wrought with sugar could be the ultimate puzzle piece to my, uh, narcolepsy, I insisted on a sleep study.

My doctor referred me. I had the study, and guess what? I wasn't getting enough sleep, but we all knew that. No, I didn't have narcolepsy, yes, I had sleep apnea, and yes, I needed to add several hours to my nightly sleep cycle. Ridiculous, I say! I'm young! I need only four hours a night! And so the routine continued, as did so many other misjudgments in my life. I was stubborn and I was righteous, I was just *sure* I knew better—that is, until my friend and NAPO colleague Val thankfully gave a seminar at our industry conference about sleep.

Current Research on Sleep

My most respected professional organizing colleague, Valentina Sgro, is an award-winning author who brings the world of professional organizing alive for readers in her novels and short stories featuring protagonist Patience Oaktree. Valentina's an attorney and a VIP in our industry, and I am always mindful of the concern she shared with me over my lack of sleep when we got together at our annual industry board meetings. Here's what she has to say about eliminating vicious sleep cycles, overeating, and underachieving.

By nature I still am an early bird. Many times I would run into the same people doing their grocery shopping at 5:00 AM. We seemed to have similar traits, such as talking into our Wi-Fi headset lodged in our ears while trying to find the coupons clipped out at midnight. For me, there were never enough hours in the day—that's why almost *all* twenty-four hours are consumed with trying to find enough stamina to finish a job at 5:00 PM or trying to talk with family members at 7:00 AM while running to catch a bus to the airport.

Then came the unbearable: because of little sleep and work overload, I would gaze adoringly at the food concessions surrounding me while trying to make a flight. That was it! Out came the Wi-Fi earpiece and in went the caramel corn and candy calling me by my first name! Every morsel was eaten in record-breaking time. With enthusiastic energy, I would board my flight, set up shop to work for five hours in the air, and then kick off my shoes to get comfy. Once settled in, so did my need to sleep—for almost the entire flight! With autopilot shut off, my mind and body were carried off by Jet Snooze.

Finally, some sleep, but at an expense that I could no longer keep up. I accomplished what I did not want to happen: sleeping at an improper time, overeating that kept my glory days as a child aflame, and not finishing my project that needed attention during that stint. How could everything that I wanted go south so quickly? The answer lies in my bed.

Sleep: Your Brain Needs to Organize Its Stuff, Too! You probably know instinctively that sleep is important. You know that babies and children need sleep to grow. You know that an injured body heals itself faster with good sleep. You know that if you don't get enough sleep, you become sluggish and cranky, and you have trouble thinking straight. That old saying, "I'll sleep on it," comes from the realization that the solution to a problem often seems to reveal itself after a good night's sleep.

What happens when you sleep? When you sleep, it is like having a well-maintained filing system. Contrary to common belief, your brain does not rest when you sleep. It is often more active than when you're awake. It's busy—busy making sure it stays organized.

What does your brain do while you get a good night's sleep? Among other things, it maintains its filing system. You know that if you have a lot of paperwork, it can quickly get out of control without a good system and maintenance. You know to buy enough filing cabinets, to sort through old files and throw out papers that were once important that you no longer need. Then you have room for newer information you need to save. And sometimes you run across papers you forgot about and you're reminded you have them. You toss some papers, like junk mail, immediately. You put some other papers in a pile and then file them later.

Your sleeping brain follows a similar process. It grows more memory capacity to hold more information. It sorts through your long-term memory and decides to forget some things that are no longer important, freeing up capacity to store newer memories for the long term. As it reviews the old memories it will keep, your brain strengthens those memories. Then it sorts the new information it received during the day. If it's not important, your brain just discards it from short-term memory. If it is important, your brain moves the information from its short-term zone to its long-term one. In other words, getting enough sleep is directly related to your brain's ability to manage information.

What happens when you don't sleep? If you don't get enough sleep, it's like letting your paperwork pile up. Your brain will become frantic, looking around for misplaced information the same way you become frantic looking around for misplaced papers if you don't take enough time to put them in their proper place. Instead of the positive chemical changes you get from a good night's sleep—the ones that improve attention, learning, and your ability to make decisions—sleep deprivation causes a lot of undesirable chemical changes in your brain. Those changes reduce your ability to concentrate, diminish your energy and performance during the day, impair memory, increase your risk of depression, deplete your immune system, grow fat rather than muscle, and accelerate aging.

A little sleep deprivation goes a long way. Cutting down on sleep just a couple of hours a night for a few weeks can cause you to lose your sense of humor without you even realizing it. More seriously, if you're getting six hours of sleep a night and have one alcoholic drink, one study showed that to be the equivalent of six alcoholic drinks if you're getting eight hours of sleep a night. In other words, just one drink can cause dangerous impairment if you are sleep deprived. (That's an extremely scary thought for parents of young adults!)

If that sounds too subjective to you, consider this statistic. In the four days after we lose an hour to switch to Daylight Saving Time, there is a 7 percent increase in accidental deaths compared to the one-week periods before and after that time. There's no downside to getting enough sleep. But, you say, you have too much to do; you'll get more sleep as soon as you catch up.

Unfortunately, that attitude is like being "penny wise and pound foolish." What you lose in time by sleeping you make up in increased productivity when you're awake. One night's sleep debt reduces the time it takes you to reach total exhaustion by 11 percent. On the other hand, sleeping one hour longer at night boosts your alertness by 25 percent. So start by convincing yourself that sleep is at least as worthwhile an activity as everything else you need to do. Put sleep on your to-do list as a high-priority item. Maybe even shift your mindset so that your day begins when you go to bed at night, and when you get up in the morning you can already cross a big eight-hour task off your list as having been successfully completed.

It all comes back to the waistline. To summarize: You've put things off, added in more things than you would have time to do in any event, and so you cut down on sleep to try to catch up. Your brain gets tired, and now, in addition to your environment being disorganized and overwhelming, your brain is disorganized and overwhelmed, too.

And, if that isn't bad enough, now studies are showing that sleep deprivation can cause weight gain as well. Sleep loss affects weight loss because it slows down your body's ability to burn calories at the same time that you begin to make unwise food choices for the sake of convenience and comfort.

If you don't feed your brain sleep, it gets cluttered, plus you eat more—and more of the wrong stuff—even as your metabolism slows down. Feed your brain sleep, and it deals with its stuff and you don't gain—maybe even lose—weight. Sleep, organization, and health. They all go together.

Today, I'm a good parent to myself. I know for sure, without a doubt, that the first breakdown in my personal health is with sleep deprivation. I still work hard and I'm probably still a bit hardheaded, but I've got the sleep thing down. My wake-up time is 5:30 AM every day, and my bedtime is 10:30 PM (it took me awhile to get comfortable with the fact that adults might need bedtimes, too). At 10:30 PM my light is off unless I have an evening event or a class or something. In that case I generally look to the next day to see where I can fit in a nap. Let's be clear—this is a planned nap, not some staggering, sleep-deprived search for a surface in which to suddenly—in the middle of everything—find a place to rest my overexhausted self, but rather a real, planned nap scheduled into my calendar.

If it's in the middle of the day, I do my best to communicate to those around me about my sleep needs, and I really take care of myself. In doing so, I do not have to reach for any goodies to keep me awake during the day and ignite the cycle of overeating.

P.S. By sleeping a full seven hours each night, I'm more productive each day than I ever was when I was staying up until 2:00 AM trying to finish what I could not complete earlier that day. Proper sleep has changed my life.

How Sleep Ties Back to Food and Gaining Weight

Johns Hopkins University reports numerous studies suggesting that people who sleep less weigh the most. Compared with people who got seven to nine hours of rest each night, people who regularly slept less than four hours nightly were 73 percent more likely to suffer from obesity. One hypothesis is that shorter sleep duration is linked with imbalances in two hormones, leptin and ghrelin. Leptin is produced by fat cells and tells the brain when to stop eating, while ghrelin, which is produced by the stomach, triggers hunger. Leptin levels decline while ghrelin levels rise in people who are not getting enough sleep.

"Sleep is no different from diet or exercise," says Carol Ash, DO, a sleep specialist in Jamesburg, New Jersey. "We know that eating

10 percent more calories a day can add fifteen-plus pounds to our frame in a year. But we fail to understand that sleeping 10 percent less carries a similar risk for weight gain." In fact, women who sleep five or fewer hours a night are one-third more likely to gain thirty-three pounds over the next sixteen years than those who get seven hours of slumber, the *American Journal of Epidemiology* reports.

According to an article written by Carolyn Richardson at www.caloriecount.about.com, "Regardless of their diet and exercise regimen, dieters lost more fat when they got more sleep." A study by the University of Chicago and the University of Wisconsin–Madison placed obese and overweight participants in two groups, one with 5.5 hours of sleep and one with 8.5 hours of sleep over a 14-day span. With the same exercise and diet during that time, those with more sleep lost more than 50 percent of their weight from fat, while the group with 5.5 hours of sleep saw only a 25 percent fat loss."

Organizing Tips for Better Sleep

By now you know me well enough to know that I will try just about any experiment or life adventure to figure my way out of a dilemma. Insomnia is no different. During the time when I was afraid to fly on planes, was fearful of bridges, and was experiencing severe anxiety attacks after the Northridge earthquake in Los Angeles, I was not able to sleep. Applying the "visioning" expertise I had learned back in gymnastics in order to complete successful and winning routines, I applied the same method to get myself to sleep. I created a sleep script. Below is a sample sleep script for you to try in case you can't shut your brain off long enough to say the letter zzzzzzz.

Dorothy the Organizer's Sleep Script

Every time I pick up this sleep script, I immediately relax. I know that as I begin to read each word, my body loosens and my brain deactivates.

I love crawling into bed because soon after I lay my head on the pillow, my breathing becomes rhythmic and I begin to feel sleepy. I will sleep amazingly well tonight and will sleep soundly every night. I love the quiet of the night, and when sounds outside occur, they do not disturb me at all. My thoughts are always on my breathing and my satisfaction about relaxing in bed. I love to sleep, and it comes easily to me. I sleep continuously though the night and I awaken with energy and happiness.

Professional organizing expert Valentina Sgro suggests the following for what to do when you really can't sleep:

The statistics are compelling, so maybe you truly are convinced on an intellectual level that skimping on sleep is a bad idea. But subconsciously that long list of overdue tasks just won't let you sleep. Or maybe you're up against a true deadline. What can you do?

1. You can use napping as a stopgap measure—a short dose of sleep so that you can refocus long enough to get something worthwhile done.

2. If you're sleep deprived, a nap will improve your performance, but not your mood. But maybe, in the short run, that's all you need. And, of course, there's the perennial favorite of those fighting to stay awake: caffeine. If ingested in the right quantities, caffeine acts as a stimulant. (Be careful, though, as too much caffeine can act as a depressant.) And while caffeine can worsen performance that involves short-term memory—so maybe it's not so good if you're cramming for an exam—caffeine will improve your performance of simple tasks that require attention rather than memory. Once you've pushed through and completed a few tasks, maybe your subconscious will reward you by relaxing enough to let you get the sleep you need.

3. What to do when you think you can't sleep? Sometimes, because you're so far behind, you think you can't sleep. There

are some good tricks to relax your brain just enough to get you started. And, as with many things, getting started is often the hardest part. Exercise often gets the body in a state where it's more receptive to sleep. Certain herbs can help, too. Lavender—just a small sachet under your pillow or in the pocket of your pajamas—can induce sleep. A cup of chamomile tea before bed can make you drowsy. If you don't like the taste of chamomile, try soaking in a warm tub of water in which you've steeped a couple of chamomile tea bags. It's extremely relaxing—and, no, it won't stain your bathtub.

4. Of course, if you find yourself already in bed and still sleepless, there's that time-honored tradition of counting sheep. It will bore both sides of your brain—the analytical side with the counting task that poses no challenge, and the visual side with the endless parade of identical sheep.

Face Overdoing It or Being Overwhelmed

Sometimes life hands us circumstances that can make us feel overwhelmed. For example, over the last five years, my family and I faced lots of harsh realities. My sister Pat was diagnosed with stage IV cancer in 2008. When she was diagnosed, we needed to make decisions as a family because it was unclear how long she had to live. I moved in to my sister's home (Mom lived there, too) and I offered to start making the mortgage payments for the house to ease my sister's financial burden. After a year, and even though I viewed this as my temporary residence, I realized I felt incredible guilt about thinking of moving back to my own place in the future. I knew that I eventually had to leave, but did not know when to move forward. I felt to move out would seem like I was deserting my sis and mom when they needed me most. Instead of declaring a move-out date, I muddled through helping with family finances, doctors' appointments, gardening, and home repairs.

I also started muddling to the freezer at two in the morning. In the middle of the night, long after the girls were asleep, I would tiptoe (à la the Grinch) down the stairs to the kitchen. I was very sly about opening and closing freezer doors and cupboard drawers without making a peep, and every once in a while a hinge would squeak. My mother, whose room was on the first floor, was lickety-split out of bed, flicking on the lights and asking, "Who's here?" Talk about feeling eight years old again. Spoon in mouth and half a pint gone, here came the questions and the lecture. I can't imagine what it's like for a parent to see her adult daughter self-destruct, and there is no good way to talk to anyone who is caught in the act of over-eating, or in the midst of another bottle-bender, or, for that matter, sitting in the middle of a hoarded-out room. Nothing they can say can shine a light in the "closed cave" we've built for ourselves—and hey—there's only enough room for one in here, so lay off, okay? I wasn't too friendly when it came to being lectured about the food I had just prepared to eat in secrecy. In fact, I wasn't nice at all. I'm sorry, Mom.

As I grew heavier, the feelings of entrapment kept me in a depressed mood. The only way out was ice cream, popcorn, potato chips, and chocolate. I think we all may know that the more you eat, the more you eat, and the less you do, the less you do. My vicious cycle was at its worst. Deep down, I knew the answer was to move out, and just like my marriage, I stayed in it far longer than was healthy for me. I wouldn't listen to my intuition, and I only heard the noise of overwhelming emotions being broadcast through my brain.

I was deeply unhappy. I spoke to my therapist, Sharma. I lamented to Nancy, Diana, Jeanette, my business partners Debby and Ken, and my new boyfriend at the time. All of them said, "Dorothy, you need to move out—the situation isn't right for you. You can't afford to keep paying the mortgage anymore. You need to thrive in your own space." I even confided in my sister Pat, who felt my pensive moods and told me to go when I was ready. Do you think that finally with her blessing I would start making my move? *No!* Instead, I kept this cycle of denial going on—until the other shoe dropped.

Once again, fate handed our family another blow. My aunt Ingrid (my mother's sister) died a painful death from cancer—she had lingered for more than seven years. She and her husband and daughter (my cousin Ruthie) resided in Florida, and Aunt Ingrid was a crucial part of our family. Now we all needed to face the fact that her daughter, Ruthie, who is physically and mentally challenged, needed a caring home upon my aunt's passing, and we agreed to fly her from Florida to Los Angeles just days after Aunt Ingrid died. My then-seventy-five-year-old mom took care of my aunt in her last days of life, and we were now facing the kind of responsibility that would deplete our hearts and souls for years to come.

It happened almost immediately. Ruthie became very sick. Between filming television shows, seeing clients, and handling media interviews, I found myself spending nights at the emergency room and days holding my mother's or Pat's hands in shock because of our situation. First, Ruthie needed her entire gall bladder removed. Then she needed to have a fibroid removed, and then she was diagnosed with uterine cancer. How is this fifty-five-year-old woman, who is developmentally age five, going to understand another surgery, chemo, and radiation? How was I going to manage my aging mother, my ailing cousin, my almost-recovered sister, and me? Who was going to pay for all this? How would we cope? Ruthie, whose mother had *just* died from cancer, instinctively knew the devastation of this disease. While we all cried together, I went back to my room and ate.

Again, we had to huddle and strategically plan out how we were going to take care of Ruthie. I refer to that time of my life as the "Three Cs: Cancer, Chemo, and Caregiving;" I was overwhelmed with more than I could bear. My sister and I took turns staying at the hospital while Ruthie convalesced. I worked twenty hours a day to make the mortgage payments, the recession was at its worst, my family seemed to be decimated by ill health, and I just couldn't keep up.

The pain and illness of chemotherapy were too much for Ruthie and us to bear. Her painful cries and nausea kept my mother up at night, and eventually kept me up, too. I was suffering watching my own mom suffer. Everywhere I turned, there was pain and overwhelming situations. Days later, I walked into a 12-step meeting. Could that meeting have been my miracle? Two weeks later, I summoned my other sister, Chris, to help us with this crisis; she arrived in an L.A. minute. One month later, I looked for and found an apartment. Two months later, I set up my own place. Four months later, Pat was in full remission. Five months later, Ruthie was healthy and back home with her father. Six months later, I broke up with my dear, sweet boyfriend of two years, and I was finally poised to put down the food and face my stuff.

Sometimes we need to be driven to the brink. With addiction, I had heard that many of us have to go to the bottom before we are desperate enough to save ourselves. I was desperate. In this case, I didn't even go to that meeting because I was wildly overweight; I went to that meeting because I needed a community of people who understood my mental obsession with food. It was there that I could finally see that my life was out of control—and for a professional organizer who seeks control in nearly all areas of her own life and helps others to achieve it, something had to change.

Today, the word "overwhelmed" is not part of my language. I can't afford to even move in the same circles that have the word "over" attached to them. Overweight, overtired, overspending, overcommitted, overworked—I can't go there. I *won't* go there. I learned all I need to know about what I coined the "O'Factor," and I can't have any of it. When I get the very first clue that I might not get proper sleep, I check my calendar the next day to see where I can insert a nap. If I want to make a purchase and don't have the money, it goes on a list and I prioritize the purchases; I no longer just buy what I want when I want it. I have also come clean: I am not a money tree. While I can loan money to others now and again, I no longer allow myself to take on mortgages I cannot afford or buy expensive chemotherapy drugs without getting a clear confirmation of my reimbursement, as was the case with my cousin. And clearly, I can no longer overwork. Being a workaholic was almost as detrimental to me as overeating; it was preventing me from having a balanced life. I am now strict with my work hours, my bedtime, and my spending, and I'm good at self-parenting. While my real parent, my mom, is still living, I would like to enjoy our time together as two adults rather than only in the midst of the parent-child relationship I was hanging on to only a few years ago.

Current Research on Being Overwhelmed

Now that you have had a taste of my life with all its overwhelming situations and emotions, let's talk about yours. Are you suffering from the O'Factor—the phenomenon of being overtired, overspending, overeating, overcommitted, and simply being downright overloaded? Chances are that if you are suffering from the O'Factor, you are having difficulty, like I was, saying no to others and difficulty in saying yes to yourself. Is this possible?

Perhaps you need to ask yourself a few questions regarding this O'Factor madness:

- Do I have a hard time saying no to others?
- Do I continuously feel like I'm letting others down?
- How much of the day am I feeling guilty?
- How often do I say yes when I really wish I had said no?

- Which people can I say no to and why do I think this is so?
- If I have a difficult time saying no, why is this?
- Do I eat or act out to avoid obligations or avoid situations?

In fact, when it comes to overdoing it, my nonstop research assistant, Gillian, hypothesized this correlation inspired by an article titled "Bargain Shopping Is 'as Good as Porn'—Study," published in the *Australian Herald Sun*:

- Overshopping: Finding bargains produces "happy hormones."
- Overcommitting: Achieving and crossing stuff off a to-do list produces "happy hormones."
- Overeating: Those carbs, sugars, and fatty foods affect the brain, and yep, more "happy hormones." This counteracts the effects of stress hormones in the body and brain *and* can create addictive behavior.

Yet when we overshop, overeat, overcommit, or get overstressed, we are *dis*tressed and depressed about our bad, out-of-control repetitive behavior, and we produce unhappy or stress hormones. We naturally and easily medicate our own depressed, anxious, and stressed brain chemistry with the "happy hormones" that foods such as sugar, carbs, and fats produce. Ergo, the O'Factor is an ever-growing domino effect basically fueled by "happy hormones" and "unhappy hormones," *and* as we gain more weight, we need a bigger hit of "happy hormones" to actually feel happy!

How Being Overwhelmed Ties Back to Food and Gaining Weight

I know that it feels good to do things for others; however, when I constantly say yes to others and don't take care of myself and put myself into a state of being overwhelmed, I unconsciously look for ways to act out. Some of us act out with food, some of us do it with cluttering, gambling, drinking, procrastinating—you name it. Bottom line: by overlooking ourselves, we seek a quick fix to substitute the self-care we did not build in for ourselves originally.

Fine, you want me to volunteer for that event? I'm going to show you! I don't have the time to volunteer. I'll do it anyway, but you have no idea how busy I am! You want me? Fine, I'll do it, but I'll tell you what, I'm gonna have a pint of ice cream as my reward afterward! How's that? I'll show you! Yeah, right, I'll show you. Two hundred pounds is what I'll show you. If only I could have graciously declined and taken care of myself, I would not have had to resent the folks out there who were asking me for another favor. While I need to say no sometimes, I can say yes other times, as long as I get to take care of myself. No food required.

Why say no, you ask? You're always going to get a lot of requests, invitations, and even demands on your time, and we all know you simply can't "add" more time to your day. Are you indentured to then suffer from the O'Factor? The answer is *no*, if you are deliberate about saying no. It may not be easy, but it is a direct road to stress relief.

Suggestions for Saying No

- Remember, saying no doesn't have to be considered selfish. When you say no to a new, incoming request, you are ensuring your own integrity by keeping your word to other commitments you've already made *and* you will have the time to enjoy doing them.
- Allowing yourself to say no allows you to try something new! Just because you've always been the secretary for the Boy Scout troop doesn't mean you have to keep doing it forever. A confident "no thanks, for this term" gives you space to pursue other new activities.
- Being a yes guy or gal all the time isn't healthy. When you enter into the O'Factor zone, you create increased stress, which

translates into sleepless nights, which forces you to consume more sugar to stay awake. More sugar begets more sugar and displaces healthy eating. All of this has us feeling more run-down, and we are at risk for getting sick.

I could have saved *years* of agony if I could have used the word *no*. No to the wrong relationships, no to stupid mistakes, no to jobs that were offered to me but weren't for me, no to the people who took advantage of my good nature. For all intents and purposes, the word *no* was like a four-letter word, banned in our household. My dad could soothe and calm the nastiest customers at the bank where he worked. A gentleman to a fault, he only wanted to please. But that same overly kind, calming exterior led to his binge eating and diabetes. Little did he realize that by saying no, he could have extended his life and created genuine happiness. One of his surviving daughters—me—also found that people pleasing was an instant claim to fame—yet also part of a devastating circular pattern of food bingeing for years to come, accompanied by more people-pleasing behavior.

In addition to saying "no" more judiciously, I noticed many of my clients were suffering from what I coined the "Self-Sufficiency Fallacy," which is a code phrase for the "I have to do it all myself!" syndrome. With all the new gadgets and software for home and office, you're expected to constantly learn new skills and do everything online. You're now travel agents booking your flights online, bankers transferring balances online, stockbrokers trading online, and designers and publishers creating birthday cards, logos, photo albums, and newsletters online. You are landscapers and decorators redesigning your homes online; you do your own faxing, accounts receivable, letter writing, and many repairs yourself.

Plus, now you get to play "border patrol" to protect your identity from hackers. You have to install firewalls and antivirus software, and you can't just throw mail and paperwork away, you have to *shred* it first! Trying to be it all, do it all, and have it all just doesn't work. We're too busy being tired, disorganized, and stressed out to live the life of our dreams!

Tackling Overwhelming Situations and Emotions

How do we stop the overwhelming madness? You see, whether it is 10:00 AM, 4:00 PM, or 7:00 PM and you are facing an overwhelming moment, situation, or event, you must stop and regroup. I think it is essential to *stop* and ask yourself, *What do I need right now?* and then revise your plan for the rest of the day or evening.

I remember a situation some years ago, when, in the middle of my own overwhelming state, I invented a system called Operation Take Control. One Friday I was driving from Los Angeles to San Diego to give a seminar on a Saturday afternoon to the Marine Corps Air Station in Miramar (I was speaking to the Marines; why else would I come up with a system called Operation Take Control?). The drive was supposed to take two and a half hours, and I made a dinner commitment with several colleagues that Friday night before the seminar in the beautiful oceanside city of Carlsbad.

The traffic, however, was bumper to bumper, and I was running late and I still needed to meet my friends for dinner, get to my hotel, finish preparing my seminar and all the props for tomorrow, and call the hospital to check on my uncle's status (he was on life support). In addition, I wanted to swim at the hotel pool, read my e-mail, pick up all of my voice mails, and get a good night's sleep.

Operation Take Control (Use This to Get Your Life Back in Order)!

Upon arriving at the restaurant in Carlsbad, I followed my Operation Take Control plan:

1. *Stop* everything!
2. Ask myself, *What do I need in this moment?* and *What is it that absolutely must get done?*
3. Meditate on it for three to five minutes.
4. Pull out a notepad. Redesign the rest of the day/evening.

Here is how it looked:

7:00 PM	Enjoy my dinner with colleagues and let them know I need to leave at 8:45 PM.
8:45 PM	Say "Good night" to my colleagues (even if they plan to stay on at the restaurant).
8:50 PM	Drive to hotel.
9:30 PM	Check into hotel.
9:45 PM	Call and check on uncle on life support.
10:00 PM	Brush teeth, pray, write down what I think I'm going to eat tomorrow.
10:15 PM	Get to bed early (so I can get up early and finish what I didn't get to).

By implementing Operation Take Control, I was able to *stop* my crazy, spiraling, out-of-control thinking and regroup. I was able to lower my stress level with meditation and organize the rest of my evening with just the "must-dos." My "must-dos" also included taking care of my health, getting a good night's sleep, and planning a healthy day of eating the following day.

In fact, because I was in traffic, I was forced to amend my schedule and just do what was absolutely necessary. In doing so, I was less hurried, got more sleep, and was infinitely better prepared to finish writing my seminar in the morning. Instead of greeting my audience with a superficial smile while digesting a 3,000-calorie breakfast of doughnuts and coffee, Operation Take Control ensured my success.

It can work for you, too. I would like to share with you one more tip when it comes to being overwhelmed. Shhhhhhhh, it's a secret. *Ask for help. Get help.*

Need an opinion? Ask for help. You don't know how to buy a car on your own? Ask for help. You can't figure out the "easy-to-install" plasma television frame? Ask for help. You don't know where to buy a reasonably priced HEPA-filter vacuum cleaner? Ask! Can't make a decision between a Mac or a PC? Ask! Are you getting the drift, my friends? The secret is: *Ask!*

Face Your Lack of Time

Not long after I had written the book *Time Efficiency Makeover* and had appeared on the *Dr. Phil* show as a time management guru, I flew to Wisconsin for one of NAPO's chapter meetings. While there, I met up with my brother and his family and my best high school pal, Andrea. Without a care in the world, I took off my watch, ignored all the clocks, and acted as if time was no issue. For once, I wanted a break from being so regimented. What I can tell you is that both my parents were on-time kind of people. Well, no, I should say "early people." To Mom and Dad, being on time meant being ten minutes early. My training was top-notch, and it was built into my system—hands down, I was an on-time kinda gal, too.

That is, except when I went to catch my plane back home from Madison to Los Angeles. Without my fear of flying to drag me down, I stood in line with everyone else waiting to get my boarding pass and check my overweight suitcase. (*Overweight suitcase? Now wait a minute. . . . Does that mean anything?* I say to myself. *If I'm overweight, does it really mean anything at all that my suitcase is not only overweight, but that I have to pay a fee? Should I read into the fact that the bag is actually advertised with a fluorescent tag marked HEAVY? Are people staring at me and wondering that, too? Oh, there goes the self-esteem thing again—why didn't I diet sooner? When I get back, I swear I'm losing this weight for good.*) Oh, to be in my head in those days—scary, very scary.

I snap out of my emotional obsession about weight and answer the airline desk clerk, "Ah, yes," I say. "Los Angeles, please—here's my reservation paperwork and my ID."

"Los Angeles?" she repeats as though I've just lost my mind.

Distractedly, I tell her, "Uh, yes."

Pointedly, she told me that the flight had left an hour ago.

What? I think to myself again. *Don't you know I'm a time management junkie? Don't you know I write books on the subject? Don't you know what time it is? Oh dear. Where's my watch? . . . . My watch! Where did I leave my watch?* (I suppose that's how most people feel when they misplace their keys.) Before I even had the chance to spin out of control, I just had to laugh at myself, and I saw a comical newspaper headline flash before me: PROFESSIONAL ORGANIZER/TIME MANAGEMENT EXPERT MISSES PLANE, LOSES TRACK OF TIME.

Admittedly, this kind of time mismanagement doesn't happen often, but I noticed the more preoccupied I was with food, the less I cared about how I looked or how late I was for appointments. And another thing, I learned that I do a little thing called "Planned Procrastination." As long as I had food to support me and keep me awake, I could wait until the last possible second to finish projects and presentations; sugar nurtured my creativity when I needed it the most—which was at the last possible second. My schedule matched my eating habits—hectic, with last-minute food snatches from drive-through windows at fast-food joints. I knew myself well enough that I would simply procrastinate to the point of no return, and I was forced absolutely to finish a project or else! I didn't just put it off each day and hope to get to it (regular procrastination); I planned mine. In fact, planned procrastination is a real term used for people like me who are just looking for another adrenaline rush.

The Case of Addictivity

Many of us are procrastinators, it's true. Also, many of us are really quite capable—heck, even really good—"starters" of projects. Love 'em! Start 'em! Don't wanna finish 'em. And then there are those very few who are excellent "stoppers." I mean those people who can start something and have the ability to stop a project or activity when called for. Still don't recognize what I'm talking about? I have found, through my own experience, that I used to have a tough time stopping certain behaviors—and I'm not just talking food here!

Have you ever found yourself on the Internet, say, Facebook, and you plan to stay on until just 10:00 PM? Then 10:00 comes and you decide, *Oh, just fifteen minutes more.* Then 10:15 arrives and you say, *Okay, just five more minutes . . .* Then 10:20 shows up and you say, *Well, I'll just finish this last post . . . or two.* Yeah, it's 11:00 and the Facebook page is still open on your computer screen! Ouch!

Perhaps this occurs for you when watching late-night TV. You just don't want to turn off that marathon of *Law & Order* or put down the latest *New York Times* bestseller. That discipline—that stopping mechanism—just seems to be "out of order," and we seem powerless over eating another handful of nuts from the can, buying another decorative item for the house, playing another video game, or trying on another outfit and risk being late for work. In addition to not being able to stop activities we've started, many of us just need to be busy all the time—just for the sake of being busy. It's like we're addicted to activity: addictivity!

In terms of my own transformation regarding my time management skills, I can proudly say that I practice the time management tips I offer. I can, however, look to my clients to see the drastic before-and-after scenarios concerning the ticking of the clock. I have thousands and thousands of clients—CEOs, busy moms, teachers, artists, dentists, dancers, celebrities, students, ranch owners, professional athletes, hoarders, and millionaires. Do you know what most of them have in common? Difficulties with time management.

America is experiencing a crisis. We are no longer just in information overload. We are in adrenal overload. Our adrenal system tells us to be ready, be alert; something is going to happen, danger, danger! Because we are living in a constant state of readiness, we are being gobbled up by a culture that values quick answers and changes that happen overnight.

As individuals it is becoming harder and harder to say no, because the technology in our lives provides more ways for others to make requests of our time and attention. Home phones, regular mail, cell phones, iPads, voice mail, e-mail, faxes, texts, and interactive television push us to add another to-do to our list rather than *subtract* something from our list. Many of my clients look me in the eye when we sit down for a consultation and ask me if I can help them just get their weekends back. It sounds simply impossible for them to even fathom having a full weekend to enjoy rather than being a slave to all the to-dos that have gone undone over the course of the week.

At this point, it may sound *im*possible . . . but it *is* possible. For this to come true, what we'll have to do first is tackle some of the obstacles. And to get at the obstacles, let me ask you some questions. Do you:

- Arrive and leave for appointments on time every day, have easy commutes, and take nice leisurely lunches?
- Have all of your calendar entries listed with a solid sense of what you're doing tomorrow and the rest of the week?
- Spend quality time with your family on a regular basis?
- Spend time with yourself to relax, meditate, and regroup?

No . . . none of these? Actually, I'm really not surprised. I know that for the most part, you *don't* have time; it has *you*! Our schedules are stuffed; we're dancing as fast as we can. We don't have to-do *lists*, we have to-do *novels*, and we're stressed out! In fact, according to the National Sleep Foundation, Americans, in general, work more and sleep less than any other culture in the world. And then there's the clutter—we have more of that, too: on the desk, the floors, in the filing cabinets, in the closets, and in the garage. Clutter is everywhere, which only adds to the stress and mismanagement of our time. It traps us. It drains our energy, and it steals our dreams.

By the end of the 1980s, we Americans had more material possessions than at any other time in history (and compared to any other place in the world). So, *more* stuff, *more* work = *less* sleep and *less* free time. I tell my clients that by getting enough sleep, organizing their clutter, and making more intentional choices about their time, they hold the passport to freedom, their own key to the kingdom. And that key is to simplify your life and commitments.

It's time to get back to the basics, to what really matters in life. In order to make more time for what you really love and take the stress out of your life, it's time to eliminate the unessential clutter, activities, and people in your life. If you can implement organizing and time management tools—and prioritize what's most important in your life—you can get rid of another reason to hit the fridge and overeat.

Current Research on Time Management and Procrastination

"Procrastinate" is a verb meaning "to put off intentionally the doing of something that *should be done*." Procrastination is as common as there are people on Earth. Everyone procrastinates at one time or another. Procrastination is a habit, not a fatal flaw. It is probably the single most common hindrance to effective time management. It takes persistence to change, but you can do it. Very simply stated, procrastination is the deliberate act of excessive postponing.

How much trouble your postponing causes depends to a large degree on the price you have to pay for that behavior.

Procrastination is the avoidance of doing a task that needs to be accomplished. This avoidance can lead to feelings of guilt, inadequacy, depression, and self-doubt. Procrastination has a high potential for painful consequences. It interferes with professional, academic, and personal success. Psychologist William Knaus estimates that 90 percent of college students procrastinate. Of these students, 25 percent are chronic procrastinators, the ones who usually end up dropping out of college.

Not a Time Management Problem

According to Joseph Ferrari, associate professor of psychology at DePaul University in Chicago, procrastination is not a time management or planning problem. Procrastinators do not differ in their ability to estimate time; however, they may be more optimistic in their ability to complete tasks. "Telling someone who procrastinates to buy a weekly planner is like telling someone with chronic depression to just cheer up," insists Dr. Ferrari.

It's a Shift in Priorities

In addition, fear can be a driving force for procrastination. For example, we may worry that we can't pay our bills next month and begin to work overtime to compensate for that financial shortfall. Suddenly, tasks at home to which we've already committed don't get done, and, sadly, we are incorrectly labeled procrastinators. A whole new pattern begins, and eventually we do fall victim to the label.

How Procrastination Works Inside Your Head

A task is a task. It is our "feeling" toward the *task* that may cause us to procrastinate. Every day we are confronted with tasks, whether writing a paper, cleaning the garage, or paying our bills. Inside our heads, we deal with feelings about the task that guide what we do. If those feelings are negative, we may put off the task. The result is that we can use our feelings to deal with the task rationally or irrationally.

The rational voice says, "I hate cleaning the garage, but because company is coming this weekend, I'd better get to it now. You never know what might come up before then." The irrational voice says, "I hate cleaning the garage and this task is just too big. We have company that is coming this weekend, but I can avoid taking them into the garage, and, really, summer is a much better time to be dealing with it."

Feelings of Inadequacy

According to Sharma Bennett, a licensed psychotherapist practicing in Los Angeles (whom you met earlier in the book as my therapist), the act of procrastination is also the act of postponing the actualization of one's potential. Fear-based, these cluttered thoughts distract one from the deeper issues of life. The continued act of procrastination can result in feelings of worthlessness and inadequacy. Let's look at the following list to see where your procrastination stumbling blocks may arise.

Managing Procrastination

"I know I can't do this." We certainly live up to our expectations. If you think that you can't do a task, you won't be able to. If you think that you are worthless, unloved, or unchangeable, you will feel depressed and unmotivated. It's time to change the phrase to "I know I can do this."

"The task is just too big." This is looking at the forest and not the trees. Analyze the project as a series of tasks and not one large one. Try to realistically figure out how long it takes to complete the subtasks (trees). Break down large projects into at least five smaller, more manageable sections and work on them one at a time.

"I can't get started." Ninety percent of getting started is showing up! The hardest part of running or working out is getting out the door. Once you get going, your heart starts pumping and you make progress. Break large projects into smaller, more manageable sections and work on them one at a time. Even when you don't feel like it, just take one tiny step—just one.

"I'm afraid I will mess this up." "The only thing we have to fear is fear itself," President Franklin Roosevelt said. You are afraid that your friends and colleagues will know that you are a failure if you mess up the assignment. You may think you are in over your head. Predicting this outcome can be immobilizing. Let's create a positive outcome.

"I don't know how to do this." If you don't speak French you won't know to *ouvrez la fenêtre* (open the window) when asked. If you lack training, skill, ability, or access to the resources to do the job, you may avoid the task completely. Seek out the knowledge of the task, and ask others if you need to.

"I need to do things perfectly." "Every time, all the time, I'm a perfectionist. I feel I should never lose," said Chris Evert-Lloyd. In this case, you may stop even before you start. Because you will settle for nothing less than perfection, you make the task more difficult than it has to be. You end up avoiding the task and procrastinating. Instead, use my favorite organizing slogan: "Avoid perfection at all costs" and finish the project. As a teacher used to say, "If you want perfection or nothing, you'll get nothing every time."

"I've never done this before." Pride comes from accomplishment. Pride and self-growth come from trying new things. Pride and self-growth increase your self-image. Positive self-image replaces fear. It is the fear of the unknown. When doing something for the first time, you have no way of knowing how well you will do. We desire comfort in familiar things, and this may delay your beginning the task.

"I can't get any work done around here." How can I prepare dinner if the kitchen isn't clean? How can I repair my motorcycle if my tools aren't in order? It's kind of tough to paint a painting on top of an existing painting. It's necessary to have a blank canvas to create your new painting. When you sit at your desk you may find yourself daydreaming, staring into space, doodling, or checking your e-mail every other minute. The reasons may be that your work area is distracting and noisy, your desk is cluttered and disorganized, or you are in areas that aren't conducive to work. Take just ten minutes and clear some space for your work.

"I have too many things to do." Living in an overwhelmed state is the new American way—not *the* way, but the American way. You aren't managing your priorities effectively. If you consider everything a priority, nothing is a priority. You must come to terms with the idea that there's just too much stuff, information, and projects. With computers at your fingertips, you are empowered to do everything from downloading your bank statements to developing and sizing your photos. Remember, just because you can doesn't mean you have to.

How Lack of Time Ties Back to Food and Gaining Weight

Many of my clients use food as a reward system, especially in the face of getting a project done on time. One of my financially successful clients, Adele, told me how she used food as a motivator. Well, she thought it was a motivator until we began our work together. She said to me, "If I get out of the house on time, then I can grab a pastry on the way to work and get to the office on time"—except the "grab a pastry" part turned into a shop fest of yummies for the office, then something for her hubby, and then some adorably decorated snacks for the kids.

A trip to the bakery and *shazzam*! Adele was late for work again!

Being late for work or any appointment summoned up feelings of guilt and shame, which didn't feel so good to Adele. She admitted to nabbing some more of the pastry bits again—this time from the precious bags of yummies earmarked for her office mates, hubby, and kids. The cycle continued.

After finishing a huge financial spreadsheet, which was due by 10:30 AM, Adele wanted to implement her reward system. She walked to the company cafeteria and ordered a white chocolate decaf mocha latte with whole milk, extra whipping cream, and two extra squirts of espresso. Zing! She was ready for more hyperfocused work until lunch. Back at her desk, Adele pumped out more reports, had a quick meeting, gobbled her lunch while she worked, and then hit the wall. Pure exhaustion. She revealed that every day at 2:00 PM she couldn't keep her eyes open. She would sit at her computer barely able to focus, and she just couldn't complete her work. Her manic morning was catching up with her, and she couldn't figure out where all the time went. "I mean, I don't even leave my desk for lunch; I just keep on working," Adele related to me with amazement.

To perk herself up, a candy bar was in order from the vending machine downstairs, which gave her enough energy to finish the afternoon. But sugar being its addictive self, the tiger was out of the cage, and when Adele got home for dinner, she wanted pasta (carbs). Because she needed to do some work at home in the evening to make up for being late earlier in the day at the office, she wanted something fast. After finishing a meal—minus a salad or vegetables—Adele attempted to complete work from earlier in the day at home—neglecting her kids, husband, and personal self-care routine. This endless cycle went on for years until Adele picked up the phone to talk to me about "time management" issues. In fact, it was the food issues that were creating this whole cycle for her. I was pretty direct: "It's time to stop stuffing your face, Adele. No more procrastination—you've got to face your stuff."

Organizing Tips for Time Management

Many of us use to-do lists. They can be very effective. For others, to-do lists can be overwhelming. You need to consider a few points to figure out what kind of a to-do list works best for you. Some of you may even function best with a "to-don't" list! Avoiding a list altogether may stamp out the anxiety you feel just looking at an endless scroll of musts and shoulds.

Are You a Morning Person or a Night Person?

I recommend first getting clear on whether you are a morning or a night person. If you are bright and cheery at sunrise, I suggest looking at your to-do list, calendar, or planner then. It's when you have the most energy, clarity, and assertiveness. If, on the other hand, you are not a morning person, do not try to "get up thirty minutes earlier" to implement this idea. Work with who you are. If you are a night person, I suggest taking fifteen minutes at the end of your evening to review and plan the next day's to-dos, appointments, or agenda.

What Is the Single Most Important Thing?

If you are the type of person who has a lot of "gotta dos" on your calendar, it's wise to take a few moments to scan the list and ask yourself, *What is my single most important task to accomplish on this list?* No matter how long or short the list is and no matter how often you add to that list, you will always have the opportunity to handle life's priorities if you ask this simple question.

How Long Does It Really Take?

Perhaps your extraordinary talent is something other than the masterful estimation of time (i.e., how long it takes to do something). Though it was one of the first lessons we learned in kindergarten, some of us may need to relearn how to tell time. Nanci

McGraw, author of *Organized for Success*, notes that most people underestimate by a factor of two to four how much time a given task will require.

If you struggle with completing tasks on time, arriving to appointments on time, or estimating how long a task or project will take for you to complete, it might be worth your while to do the DTO (Dorothy The Organizer) Reality Check. Bottom line: If you want to get realistic about how long it really takes to accomplish a task for yourself, simply double the amount of time you think it will take to do. As a start, review the following table:

DTO Reality Check

Task	How Long	Double the Time
Call my girlfriend	15 minutes	30 minutes
Make and eat breakfast	12 minutes	24 minutes
Drive to my Friday morning meeting	35 minutes	70 minutes
Pick up kids from soccer	20 minutes	40 minutes

While this exercise may seem like we're stretching it a bit, if you dare to try it, you will see that the "double the time" method is fairly accurate. You see, by doubling the time, it actually helps you to account for those unexplained minutes in time that magically disappear. It's true you may talk to your girlfriend for only fifteen minutes, but if you have call waiting, you may wind up taking an extra call while she's on the phone, thereby increasing the overall time you're talking to her. Also, it probably is just a twenty-minute drive to pick up the kids from soccer, but we forget to include the stop for gas on the way to the soccer field and dropping off an extra child as a favor to another soccer mom on the way home.

For those of you who struggle with time estimation, this is a quick and easy format for practicing a new way of thinking when it comes to time. Using the simple format of doubling the time you think it will take you to complete a task or project will help you to avoid speeding tickets, missed appointments, and displacing important events in the day—one of them being taking care of *you*.

It's an Alarming Situation

One other quick tip in terms of managing your time: make friends with your mobile phone's alarm clock, and I don't mean just for waking up in the morning. These wacky widgets are chock-full of crazy ringtones and options galore. You can get alarms that repeat every night at 8:45 so you know it's time to pack your lunch and lay out your clothes for tomorrow. You can set the reminder alarm prior to a conference call or an important appointment to ensure you don't miss it but have time to prepare for the call and dial in the number without being late.

Setting a time to tell you and your kids "you've got fifteen more minutes before the car leaves in the morning" is a great training tool—and requires no screaming. Once you teach your family to listen for the alarm, and everyone understands the consequences of ignoring the alarm, it will be a rare experience when you have to say, "That's it, if you're not in the car in two minutes, I'm leaving without you!" Use technology to your advantage when you can. It can be a brilliant answer to life's little frustrations.

Emergency Time Management Tip

If you need to figure out "how to organize your time right now," try this quick little tip. For some of us, our days are so jam-packed with noise, we can't even hear ourselves think—people talking to us, radios blaring, advertising messages over the intercom in stores, nonstop television. It's simple: If you want a better-organized day, stop right now. Spend one to five minutes quietly with as little noise around you as possible. Ask yourself, *Really, what's the next right action I need to take?* Then sit quietly and breathe. The answers do come and you will accomplish what you need to do. Give yourself a break and lower your blood pressure! Go get 'em!

Organizing Tips for Addictivity

Video games, social media, television, shopping, eating, and so on can take up a lot of time that we can use productively, and the lack of exercise is not healthy. Make time to steer yourself away from some of these addictive, sedentary behaviors with more stimulating and interesting activities.

- Set boundaries for these addictive pleasures. Use a timer, for example.
- Show up ready to take a stand and battle it out a bit—not just for yourself, but for others, too.
- Enlist a "bookend" partner to whom you can be accountable. Agree to call your partner at the end of your video game or Facebook session.
- Use the "one for you and one for me" approach. Switch out your addictive obsession with other options, such as outdoor activities, clubs, and hobbies.
- Be prepared. If you really want to manage your addictivity, be sure your "other activity" items are ready for use. Make sure your putter and golf balls are accessible, make sure your sketch pad has clean pages in it, and make sure your bike doesn't have a flat.
- Get honest with yourself. If the addictivity is interfering with doctors' appointments, paying bills, sleep cycles, or relationships, it's time to seek professional help.

Face Your Lack of Finances

Much earlier in my life, I had the "What do you mean I'm overdrawn? I still have more checks in my checkbook" point of view. This horrified my dad, who was the beloved town banker back home in Wisconsin. While I was in college, and before he passed away, my dad would monitor my accounts regularly and see that I had visited an ATM and withdrawn another wad of cash. I never knew it, but he would then deposit cash into my account and—miraculously!— when I went to the ATM the next day (knowing I had no money), I would still ask it for cash and it would magically appear! Now I know why.

What a loving thing for a dad to do—and enabling, too. Since the age of twelve, I worked hard: babysitting, running a little gymnastics center out of my parents' home when I was fifteen, becoming a receptionist at a law firm at sixteen, and so on. I certainly did understand what it took to make a buck. Spending it, though? That was a problem. I didn't care about the consequences; I wanted what I wanted when I wanted it. Come to think of it, I was that way with food, too.

As I reflected, I took a closer look at my own history and began to correct both my binge eating and binge spending. Indeed, there was a strong correlation. Staggering dollars' worth of daily receipts from Starbucks, Coffee Bean, yogurt joints, and Chinese takeout were being replaced with a disciplined way of eating, sleeping, working, and spending.

Since then, all of the debt my ex-husband incurred has been paid off and I've developed a new relationship to money. Oh sure, with the help of Tony Robbins, Landmark Education, and Mark Victor Hansen's books *The One-Minute Millionaire* and *Cash in a Flash*, I experimented with all sorts of new ideas:

- I tried actor Jim Carrey's idea about writing a $1 million check to myself and posting it on my wall to see every day as inspiration.
- I wrote scripts saying I could be brilliant about money, that I could attract money easily, that I am magnetic around money, and I am a money mogul.
- I donned my artist costume and created vision boards about being on the verge of living a millionaire's life—complete with pictures of luxurious travel destinations and what my house on the oceanfront cliffs looks like.
- I would go to sleep telling myself I never have to worry about money. I began to articulate all of the subtle programming I created in my mind. I got clear on all the new thoughts I could have about money.
- I also asked myself if my whole identity was wrapped up in money. What if making money was fun?

With all the food out of the way, I had the time and interest to begin looking at other aspects of my life, including my finances and my future. I also became more philanthropic. I looked further than myself and gave money to those in need. All of this practice concerning money allowed me to confidently declare my value as a professional organizing expert. The convergence of all of these activities completely redefined my ease around money. Just one small step is all it takes. Just one.

Current Research on Money

My friend Timolin Langin, aka "Timmie The Teacher," is a veteran teacher, real estate developer, and world traveler, has roots in a small town in Mississippi. There, a generation of relatives with a "mother wit" for financial success taught her how humble earnings could yield a fiscal life stable enough to support all of her dreams, travel, and interests. She writes,

If the love of money is the root of all evil, then could emotional spending be the root of all financial woes? Emotional spending, sometimes called retail therapy, refers to the belief that we can somehow spend our way to feeling good. Buying something seems like a way of soothing feelings of anger, guilt, depression, sadness, low self-esteem, fear, doubt, insecurity, and anxiety. Advertisers try to convince us that a product or service can bring us joy, confidence, status, and sexual desirability. Shopping may seem like a kind of therapy since it helps you take your mind off your problems or feelings for a moment, a temporary and sometimes financially devastating form of escape. Often, after the shopping spree ends, our uncomfortable or painful feelings soon return.

Advertisers are aware of our needs and desires to feel good, to feel special or popular, and they spend millions of dollars to encourage us to buy products or seek retail therapy. The subtle message is that acquiring these things will somehow meet our needs and we magically become well as a result. We will in an instant become beautiful, desirable, appealing. You can be "hot," as my students would say, if you wear the same lipstick as your favorite model or drive the newest sports car.

Emotional spending makes us feel popular and special within our own community. There seems to be this growing belief that we are not enough or we don't measure up in and of ourselves, and somehow if we spend more, then we will become more. If we drive the same car as our neighbor or a more expensive one, then somehow we have suddenly arrived. Advertisers gain from our retail therapy, but we the consumers lose a lot: money, dignity, and peace of mind.

Then there is the other aspect of emotional spending. A seductive aspect of retail therapy is that it appears to be fun. We are in huge, busy places with lots of people, feeling powerful, taking home boxes and bags of goodies. Let's face it; some of us just like to shop. Buying is fun; it is entertaining, and it is a way to impress our friends and keep up with our neighbors. Our neighbor bought a new SUV, so we buy a new SUV. Our friend bought a designer bag, so we buy a designer bag. Being financially competitive with others is a big reason for emotional spending. We are comparing ourselves to others and being envious and desirous of what they have, even when we know we can't afford it.

Now I am not advocating vows of poverty or a life of deprivation where you live without everything you want. I am, however, a huge fan of enjoying life while being good money managers. I just believe it is possible to balance pleasure and financial responsibility. I have been teaching financial workshops throughout Southern California for emotional spenders who have difficulty controlling their shopping behaviors and managing their money.

I have found that for many emotional spenders—people who are treating their feelings by acquiring things laden with symbolic value rather than stocking their shelves with necessities—the "hit" of buying disappears quickly but the money is gone permanently. Yet, in search of a "fix," they return to buying again and again, often sinking into serious debt. Like the alcoholic with a drink, the shopping "hit" of the emotional spender doesn't last long. As time passes, it takes more clothes, more purses, and more stuff to satisfy the emotional need. Eventually, you are forced to face the budgetary consequences of retail therapy.

Your debt may start to increase and the bill collection companies may start calling. Now you are faced with the responsibility of emotional spending. The shopping bills are due and so are the bills for the essentials of food, utilities, and shelter. Emotional spenders often find they acquired luxuries and skimped on necessities. Now family life is no longer wonderful. Studies reveal that over 50 percent of all marriages end in divorce, and finance matters or money problems are frequently cited as the number-one reason for these breakups.

Arguments ensue over spending habits, paying bills, and differing approaches to savings. Couples have difficulty resolving these differences and decide it's best to end the marriage. Single people are affected in that they too find it difficult to pay for the basic necessities of food, clothing, and shelter. Like many alcoholics, many emotional spenders do not recognize they've got a problem until things go haywire. Then feelings of guilt, inadequacy, or fear or sadness kick in. The state of euphoria that accompanied the purchase is now bringing you to new lows as the high is waning and the consequences of your spending decisions become apparent. So, like the alcoholic, the emotional spender wakes up with a hangover or what I like to sometimes call a "shopover" and begins to face the wreckage caused by retail therapy.

How Money Ties Back to Food and Gaining Weight

Often we loan others money or rescue them from their own bad choices and we are out the money we loaned, and it builds resentment toward them (let's eat) and anger directed toward ourselves (more food please, I'm feeling uncomfortable). We must treat our grown siblings, kids, friends, and parents like adults.

It is amazing that once I had my weight under control, I could see the dim but growing light in the distance. I was *done*—not only with any "diets" but also with my yo-yo spending sprees. As I reined in my financial recovery by paying down my ex-husband's debt (six felony counts plus extraordinary legal bills will do you in), the *freedom* of no credit card payments or monthly car installments was just as liberating as the freedom of taking off the pounds.

Dorothy the Organizer's Four Ways in Which Debt Can Help You Lose Weight (or Vice Versa)

1. **Start small and keep it regular.** Whether you are paying off a loan or starting a savings account, it doesn't matter how small the amount; it only matters that you do it. So it goes with losing weight and exercising. Make small changes regarding your food and keep it regular. Start walking for ten minutes a day and keep it regular. Drink an extra glass of water and keep it regular. Small changes pay off.

2. **Budget the outgoing and the incoming.** When you want to get a handle on your debt, you need to write down all of your expenditures and any incoming cash. Writing down your financial figures gives you a very real picture of what's going on in terms of your daily cash flow. It's the unforgotten ATM purchases and quick cash outlays that have you wondering where your money went. Writing down what you eat serves you in the same way. Keeping track of what you eat keeps you honest. Writing down the food you intend to eat for the day, in advance, takes you even one step closer to your weight-loss wishes and stamps out any thoughts about how those extra pounds jumped onto your bathroom scale.

3. **Communicate if it's not working.** Try as we might to be vigilant about paying down a debt, some months we may not have enough money to match our intentions. What do you do when you know you're struggling to make a payment? You reach out and communicate with the lender and share what's going on. By being in communication, you can usually control the damage. Similarly, if you're trying to lose weight and struggling with cravings, pick up the phone and communicate! Tell someone what's going on. Share your feelings and

experience. Guess what? By being in communication, you can usually control the damage.

4. **Celebrate sensibly.** Congratulations! You've just paid off your car loan. Wahoo! Here's what not to do: do not go out and purchase something to celebrate! We wouldn't suggest that an alcoholic toast with champagne after achieving a year of sobriety, so if you have reached a weight-loss goal, be sure to have a sensible reward system in place—something other than food. A massage, a walk along a quiet stream, or dancing with friends are sensible choices.

Organizing Tips for Finances

Solutions from Timolin Langin begin first with admitting you have a problem in the same way an alcoholic must admit she is unable to manage alcohol consumption: "I am a shopaholic. I spend money to make me feel good." It really is that simple. She writes,

> As a finance coach, the first thing I tell my clients is that you have to separate your feelings from your spending. The emotions you have and the purchases you make are two different things. And an impulse to purchase something you feel you want right now is very different from the purchase of a necessity like your week's groceries or the paying of your mortgage. You have to be able to distinguish between the "must-haves" and the things you can go without for now. I am not a fan of self-deprivation, but I do suggest going on a spending freeze of the nonessentials for a while until financial and emotional sobriety becomes a habit. To make good decisions when managing your money, and to curb emotional spending, I highly recommend the following six tips: create a budget, create affirmations, do something that makes you feel good, turn off your television, know your triggers, and pay cash.
>
> **Create a budget.** A budget is the dreaded "B" word that can be

intimidating at first. However, it is just a flexible, mindful plan for both short-term and long-term spending, saving, and goal setting. A budget simply requires looking at your income and expenses and then devising a plan to pay off all credit card debt and reduce the consumption of unnecessary goods and services. It also changes as your financial outlook changes. I highly recommend a four-step budget plan based on the following allocations:

- 10 percent give back
- 50 percent to needs
- 20 percent to savings
- 20 percent to elimination of debt, particularly credit cards

Ten percent of resources is designated to give back—be it to your church, synagogue, or charity, depending on your beliefs. I know giving is not a popular strategy to curbing emotional spending and building wealth, but it is one that I've used to create a good life. It is based on the understanding that God, the Universe, or a Source exists that is vastly bigger than us and operates beyond our limited boundaries, and it wants to bring abundance into our finances and every area of our lives. Perhaps you could come to think of giving back as the best and truest kind of "emotional spending"—and be sure to express your gratitude for what you have and share your good fortune with others—and in due season your financial assets will increase.

Fifty percent of your household salary is allocated to needs: food, health, and shelter. However, in my workshops I teach you ways to reduce that percentage. I also suggest allocating 20 percent of your income to savings (personal, emergency, and retirement). The last 20 percent is for elimination of credit card debt. I highly recommend the next step as a means of self-encouragement and staying committed to your budget, and reducing emotional spending.

Create affirmations. I believe that there is power in our words and thoughts. I believe you have the power to change your spending habits and financial practices in general by establishing a connection with something deep within you and believing that it is possible to overcome the obstacle of emotional spending. For example, in financial workshops I encourage an emotional spender to create a vision board with words and pictures of their desired lifestyle.

I also believe we are not to walk this earth alone and that we need a partner. I highly recommend getting what I call an accountability partner, someone whom you trust and can talk to at least once a week and call when the urge to splurge hits. Sometimes we simply need to be reminded that we are wonderful, beautiful, and enough right now, in our current state, and an accountability partner can be another valuable source of powerful words and reminder of the pictures on your vision board.

Do something that makes you feel good. Eating foods that are wholesome, exercising regularly, and getting enough sleep are behaviors that affect your feelings in positive ways, leading to good decision-making and reduction of emotional spending. Walks on the beach, conversations with loved ones, and reading a good book are excellent ways to make yourself feel better without using your credit card.

Turn off your television. Television creates a subconscious need for desire. Advertisers always tell you to spend, spend, and spend. And many things advertised are either unwholesome, like fast food, or luxuries and status symbols or other kinds of "hits" to ease our psychic and physical pains. One seldom sees fruit, meditation, or nice walks advertised.

Know your triggers and do not shop. When you are feeling sad, insecure, anxious, or stressed, don't go to a store and don't go to an online shopping site—another whole realm of hazard for addicted shoppers today. You are more likely to spend money to soothe these feelings, and when they have subsided you realize you spent money on something you cannot afford. Affirmations are most helpful here; sweat it out by jogging or walking, meditate, talk to your accountability partner, and find someone you can help. If you are consistent, the feelings will subside and eventually go away.

Pay cash. Paying with cash is a great way to stick to your budget and curb emotional spending. It encourages you to spend less, because it eliminates what I like to call mindless spending. When you pay cash for a product or service, you feel the power of that purchase immediately, and it forces you to ask, "Is this something I really want or need?" You experience buyer's remorse even before you complete the purchase and have your "shopover" while in the store and decide you can live without it.

These six positive behavior changes will get you a long way down the road to fiscal responsibility and sobriety in the use of your own money. If you utilize these strategies and still find yourself struggling with emotional spending, then it may be time for you to get formal and individualized education via a finance coach or counselor. As an educator, I truly believe that financial knowledge is power, a power that changes lives for the better. Paying conscious and careful attention to our own money is one skill not usually taught in schools. Yet how we manage our money influences our entire lives, from where we live to the amount we pay for our home and how much peace of mind we have.

There is an element of emotional spending in all spending, including spending on basic necessities. As human beings, we all have a desire to feel safe, secure, special, and satisfied. The acquisition of things fulfills an emotional need that is common to all.

Face Your Isolation and
Lack of Community Support

As a child, I liked to play with dolls by myself rather than hang out with the gang down the street. In school I preferred doing individual book reports alone rather than participate in group projects. As an athlete I gravitated toward individual sports, like gymnastics and track, rather than team sports. In my career, I excelled in the world of entrepreneurship rather than a traditional corporate setting. I belonged to 4-H, Girl Scouts, the Chamber of Commerce, the National Association of Professional Organizers, and many, many more groups, but it was always a struggle for me to function easily in a group setting. My family was relatively small, and I just didn't have the experience of group support in terms of ideas, projects, or life itself.

Here is what's cool about the *new* me, though. I ask for help! *Ta-da!* (Applause, please.) I just want to run around calling friends and neighbors, handing out flowers and pretty pens to celebrate! It's so unlike me, but I'm doing it. Writing this book is one example. Don't get me wrong: When I decided to write this book, my first thought was to write it myself. The minute that the "I'll write it myself" thought came into my brain, however, I knew, *Dorothy, you must do the opposite. Don't isolate. Build your community. Get others involved. Enhance your conversation. Give your readers some options and different writing styles. Share your life and projects. Work with others. Have fun. Don't do it alone.* Indeed, this book is a collaboration with other experts. This fabulous experiment taught me a few things:

1. Wow, I know some really great people who love and support me!
2. Working with others reduces my stress level.
3. I feel like I belong and I don't have to "do" life or projects alone.

And here's the really great part: When I feel loved, reduce my stress level, and feel like I belong, I don't have the urge to eat! *Ta-da* again! . . . this time with a tiara on my head (and a great big thank-you to everyone who contributed or supported me with this book).

Current Research
on Community Support

Our lack of community is intensely painful.
A TV talk show is not community.
A couple of hours in a church pew each Sabbath
is not community. A multinational corporation
is neither a human nor a community, and in the sweatshops,
defiled agribusiness fields, genetic mutation labs,
ecological dead zones, the inhumanity is showing.
Without genuine spiritual community, life becomes
a struggle so lonely and grim that even Hillary Clinton
has admitted "it takes a village."

—*David James Duncan*

A recent documentary produced and directed by Roko Belic proves the point that *connecting with close, supportive friends and family/community* is one of the main pillars for an individual's happiness. The movie *Happy* is more than just a movie, but rather a movement. In a November 7, 2012, blog post reviewing the documentary for the Care2 Make a Difference website (www.care2.com), Aimee Dansereau wrote, "The happiest people are those who focus their time and energy on close, supportive friends and family, and community. People who are happy tend to live longer. And there's nowhere in the world with more people who live over the age of 100 than in Okinawa, Japan. Okinawa is a close-knit society. Their traditions and community activities keep the people connecting with one another. For instance, they have a band that plays in a different village every Friday night. Everyone in the village, from young to old, comes out to see it."

How a Lack of Support and Isolation Tie Back to Food and Gaining Weight

It has been my experience that because I was determined to go at life alone, I used food as my quiet companion. But food did not supply me with any answer—just higher numbers on the bathroom scale. And the heavier I got, the less likely I was to make connections with anyone—friends, family, or new acquaintances.

According to John Cacioppo, a solid guarantee for a long, healthy life is the connections you make and maintain with other people. John Cacioppo is a neuroscientist at the University of Chicago who coauthored the book *Loneliness: Human Nature and the Need for Social Connection*. Writer Nancy Shute interviewed Cacioppo for *U.S. News and World Report* and reported, "Loneliness shows up in measurements of stress hormones, immune function, and cardiovascular function. Lonely adults consume more alcohol and get less exercise than those who are not lonely. Their diet is higher in fat, their sleep is less efficient, and they report more daytime fatigue. Loneliness also disrupts the regulation of cellular processes deep within the body, predisposing us to premature aging."

Bingo. I was headed down that path for sure. My joints ached. I slept poorly and exercised little. My diet was higher in fat, and I felt twenty years older than I actually was. While I think my isolation was born out of becoming overweight, I believe that one of the keys to my freedom was connecting with others again.

Organizing Tips for Isolation and Lack of Community

Do you know where to seek community support? Notice I didn't ask *if* you wanted community support, because the answer is usually, "No, thanks." Most of us actually do know how to eat healthily and take steps for improved fitness; however, dealing with our stuffed-down feelings can be quite an effort. Here are four ideas to get you connected again:

1. **Enlist a friend.** Think about your friends and family and seek out someone in the tribe who is looking to buddy up, too. Whether it's an accountability partner to begin decluttering projects or a meeting three times a week with a walking buddy, it's important to have a confidant with whom you can discuss your feelings. A simple four-minute phone call each day to a couple of friends (two minutes per person) can allow you to spout out your intentions for the day and feel as though you've got the support you need to make it happen.

2. **Meet with a professional.** Therapists, counselors, family doctors, and members of your local clergy are great resources for building community. These folks have the credentials and experience to help you find a group that is right for you. If you are overweight or the clutter is building again, you probably know that there is usually another concern underlying the excess around you. Furthermore, these professionals are trained to listen, understand, and confidentially help you resolve problems.

3. **Reach out online.** The Internet provides us with all sorts of meet-up groups and communities for weight loss, hiking, dating, dancing, and more. Going online can be a great source of strength and support. It's also a quick way to find other people who share your interests and similar schedules. If you decide to join a local group online, most often you can meet your new community soon after in a safe and healthy way. Once together, you can engage individually with others who may be experiencing the same emotions you are. The support can be profound.

4. **Attend a meeting.** For some of us, an in-person meeting is the perfect answer. Attending a support group or meeting allows for a regular, dependable routine. The more you attend, the

closer you become to other members in the group, thereby increasing the feeling of belonging. Facilitators at meetings are primed with ideas and tips to share and implement, whether you're trying to give up smoking, pay down debt, or lose weight. Twelve-step meetings are very effective.

Face Your Lack of Spirituality

Part of my commitment to my new life was to develop an understanding of a Higher Source that I could relate to. I always saw the Source, a Universal Power, or God as religion and not as a private source of strength meant just for me. I was perplexed and resistant. Decide how you can create your own guiding spirit? Your own concept of God? No kidding? You mean, we can decide for ourselves? Yes, you can! I did, and I'll share mine.

It is here, though, that I would like to acknowledge the many people who already have a relationship with God or their own religion. That is simply perfect. You may be all set and may not need to read this section whatsoever. There are some of us out here, however, who may still be confused, feel abandoned, have given up, or have never had the inspiration to consider a Higher Power for themselves. My personal experience suggests that, yes, you can find an entity that's bigger than yourself to provide you strength and hope each day.

It seems to be a "little out there," but I worked at developing my own God concept, and here it is: My spiritual guide is an energy force similar to that of quantum physics. My spiritual guide resembles a cloudlike puff that has a *Wizard of Oz*, fairy tale–type voice that spits out wise advice and gives me guidance and the feeling of protection. This spiritual guide (some of you may call this "God" or a "Higher Power") is accepting, loving, and healing. I know with this spiritual concept that I don't need to be perfect, I get to feel sane and serene whenever I take time out to pray, and I am accepted as I am, wherever I am. Yep, I created this whole vision of my spiritual guide.

It may seem silly to some, but it was the agonizingly misplaced piece in my life—and it was the *Who Wants to Be a Millionaire?*'s final answer to my overeating conundrum.

I now meditate for thirty minutes in the morning and pray daily. I feel at home in any temple, church, or mountaintop vista. I have a guiding spirituality that works—and keeps me from stuffing my face—and I am full of gratitude.

Current Research on Spirituality

In terms of using "gratitude" as a means for fulfilling one's spiritual practice, our in-house Zen master, Gillian Drake, uncovered research by Professors Lyubomirsky, Sheldon, and Schkade that suggests that our level of happiness is 50 percent genetics, 40 percent intention, and 10 percent circumstantial. She writes,

> The University of California, Davis (UC Davis), has a whole laboratory dedicated to the study of gratitude practice, and in 2012 the John Templeton Foundation awarded it a $5.9 million grant for a project titled "Expanding the Science and Practice of Gratitude." Researcher Dr. Robert Emmons, who heads up the lab at UC Davis, has revealed that people who conduct certain gratitude exercises are healthier and feel better about their lives, make more progress toward goals, and are more optimistic.[1]
>
> It seems that with gratitude practice, troublesome thoughts pop up less frequently and with less intensity, which suggests that gratitude may enhance emotional healing. Another researcher in the field, Professor Watkins, speculates that "thankfulness" helps the brain fully process events, and that grateful people achieve closure by making sense of negative events so that they mesh with a generally positive outlook. It may feel strange at first, but you can be grateful about many things—an easy ride home on the freeway, landing a new client, the kind act of a neighbor or friend. But most important

are the things that we often take for granted, like good health, our family, and our homes.

Just fake it until you can make it! Once you start saying "thank you," your mind will automatically find more reasons for you to be thankful. Thankfulness can help you see that you're loved and cared for. It can literally bolster your self-esteem because you realize that people care enough about you to do things for you. The benefits of practicing gratitude are numerous: you'll stop focusing on what you don't have, such as material objects or bad experiences, which can in turn reduce the number of negative emotions you experience, such as envy or nagging. Gratitude literally encourages positive focus, thus promoting more positive emotions, such as appreciation and love.

With her previous massage practice, I see Gillian Drake as a bit of a spiritual guide herself. Drake also takes on the topic of meditation and asks what meditation can do for us.

One medical dictionary defines meditation as "a practice of concentrated focus upon a sound, object, visualization, the breath, movement, or attention itself in order to increase awareness of the present moment, reduce stress, promote relaxation, and enhance personal and spiritual growth." *Webster's* more simply says, "Continued or extended thought; contemplation: the act or process of spending time in quiet thought."

To different folks, meditation means different things: deep breathing, quiet time, jogging, knitting, yoga, mantras, dancing. These mindful actions might all be construed as meditative and relaxing: ways to refocus the mind that can unwind and de-stress. And although some think of meditation as a religious or spiritual practice, in the last decade the Dalai Lama has teamed up with renowned doctors and scientists to try to prove that "mindfulness" (aka meditation) is a valuable tool that we should even be teaching to our kids to enhance their attention and focus, memory, self-acceptance, self-management skills, and self-understanding.

But it's not just a way to relax or to "connect" with your higher self: a researcher at Brigham and Women's Hospital, David Vago, has identified eight different cognitive functions that activate and develop in the brain during mindfulness practice. These cognitive functions exist as part of a framework for the development of self-regulation, self-awareness, and self-transcendence (SART).[2]

In a 2012 article published by UCLA Newsroom, it was revealed that meditation actually thickens the brain and improves cell connectivity. The UCLA Laboratory of Neuro Imaging (LONI) researchers discovered that long-term meditators have larger amounts of gyrification or "folding" of the cortex, which may allow the brain to process information faster than people who do not meditate. Among other functions, this plays a key role in memory, attention, thought, and consciousness. Presumably then, the more folding that occurs, the better the brain is at processing information, making decisions, forming memories, and so forth.[3]

Another medical researcher, Robert E. Herron, PhD, has conducted various studies on Transcendental Meditation, and he believes it could greatly reduce the average person's medical expenses. In fact, in light of evidence that chronic stress can weaken the immune system, which in turn can increase vulnerability to a wide range of physical and mental disorders and diseases, many medical practitioners recommend mindfulness to their patients on a regular basis. And it is already widely used not only to treat stress but also chronic pain, anxiety, depression, borderline personality disorder, eating disorders, and addiction.[4]

It is the Dalai Lama's hope that by teaching mindfulness to our children from an early age, we will furnish them with a tool that will help them cope more easily and instinctively with stressful situations—be they examinations, competitions, conflicts, or other emotional traumas. And it seems the benefits are astounding!

For the past three years, neuroscientist Richard Davidson, author of *The Emotional Life of Your Brain* and founder of the Center for Investigating Healthy Minds, has been starting programs in schools in Vancouver and, more recently, in Madison, Wisconsin.[5] The techniques used with children as young as four years old are quite simple. To improve a child's ability to pay attention—and also improve their studying abilities—a stone is put on a child's stomach, and they learn to focus on their breathing as the stone goes up and down. Research has also been performed with teenagers by asking them to visualize a loved one suffering followed by a thought that they be relieved of that suffering. This exercise has also been shown to produce meaningful changes in the brain and behavior. So overall, meditation or mindfulness shows pretty impressive results: improving the ability of children and adults to focus, learn, and manage their behavior and empathic responses while reducing stress improves overall well-being.

How Spirituality Ties Back to Food and Gaining Weight

Do you sometimes find yourself halfway through a bag of potato chips or packet of cookies before you realize you are even eating them? What's on your mind when you're eating? Are you really hungry? Do you really need food? Or are you experiencing anger, anxiety, disappointment, or panic? When emotions start to percolate inside, we can often literally feel nauseated or like we might explode: we fear being exposed by their "great escape." Those bubbling, churning emotions in our core can cause us to feel out of control and overwhelmed, and it's all too easy to *swallow* them down in order to regain composure or maintain balance, but at what cost? Stuffing down your emotions—mindlessly eating to keep emotions down inside us instead of dealing with them—is a common problem.

"Be as nice as pie; swallow your pride; eat your heart out; eat humble pie; follow your gut feeling" are just a few emotional/food idioms. Emotions can play a huge role in how much and how often we stuff our faces. Similarly, buried emotions or traumatic memories associated with accumulated physical stuff can cause us not to want to face our stuff. Everyone has different tolerance levels for stress and adrenaline, and a condition called "anxiety sensitization" can affect the way different people respond to stress. What one person perceives as a tummy-tingling, exciting high, another might interpret as nervous butterflies in their gut, and yet another might actually feel so anxious they become nauseated.

Anger is an emotion that is felt so strongly in the gut it actually can be misinterpreted as hunger! Depression can cause overeating, and the overeating can in turn cause more depression, creating an emotional roller coaster. People pleasers may overeat because they're very critical of themselves, they want approval, and everyone else's well-being is more important than their own. Loneliness can cause people to use food as a substitute for relationships.

Boredom can lead us to seek quick gratification from high-fat, high-sugar, and high-calorie foods. And anxiety, fear, or stress may cause us to seek comforting foods such as a bowl of pasta or ice cream. It is better not to use food as a way to cope with unpleasant emotions but rather find new ways of nurturing yourself to feel better.[6]

So how can meditation or mindfulness help you with achieving and maintaining your optimum weight? Understanding why we eat too much or not enough can help explain and change a bad emotion/food-coping mechanism.

For many people, eating fast means eating more. We've all heard that it takes twenty minutes or so for the message to get from your stomach to your brain when you are actually full. Mindful eating accomplishes many things: it is a way to slow down, to become more aware of when we have eaten enough, to take a closer look at what we're craving, and to wake us up as to why we're craving it. Harvard nutritionist Dr. Lilian Cheung has devoted herself to studying the

benefits of mindful eating and is passionately encouraging corporations and healthcare providers to try it. Google encourages a mindful lunch hour, and self-help gurus like Oprah Winfrey and Kathy
Freston have become cheerleaders for the practice.

It's not easy, so be kind to yourself. You may not be able to do
it every time you eat, but try it at least once a day for the first five
minutes of your meal and grow from there. Mindful eating could be
as simple as acknowledging that you are mindlessly eating a burrito
and driving at the same time. It's a gradual process that takes practice, but the next time you find yourself reaching for your favorite
snack, if you take a few breaths and open your mind to get in touch
with your cravings, you may be able to become more aware of your
emotional eating habits.

Organizing Tips for Spirituality

In Candi Paull's book *Checklist for Life for Women* (there's one for
men, too), each page is filled with real-time ideas on how to build a
relationship with God. If this is an area of life where you would like
to grow, perhaps some suggestions from the hundreds of ideas in the
Checklist book will start the ball rolling. Here are just ten:

1. Set aside five minutes to pray for guidance from a
   Higher Power about a specific situation that troubles you.
2. Look in the mirror and see yourself as someone lovable.
3. Look for the lesson in each detour, delay, and
   unexpected delight.
4. Listen for guidance and ask a Higher Power to help
   you make the right choices.
5. Be open to new ideas and new ways of doing things.
6. Know that your prayers will be answered for your
   highest good.

7. Be an answer to someone else's prayer with a generous gift of help.
8. Go for a walk in nature and bring home an interesting rock or leaf to remind you that God has many creative and beautiful ways to accomplish divine purposes in your life.
9. Be compassionate to others who may be lonely.
10. Mark out some time in your daily calendar for "life-appreciation breaks."

Rick Warren, often called America's most influential spiritual leader, wrote the book *The Purpose Driven Life*. In it, he quotes the Bible, which says, "Do not act thoughtlessly, but try to find out and do whatever the Lord wants you to." Warren stresses to his readers not to let another day go by, and start finding out and clarifying what God intends for you to be and do. Warren suggests,

1. Begin by assessing your gifts and abilities. Take a long look at what you are good at and what you're not good at. Make a list and ask others for their opinion. Spiritual gifts and natural abilities are always confirmed by others.
2. Consider your heart and your personality. Ask yourself questions: What do I really enjoy doing most? What am I doing when I lose track of time? Do I like routine or variety? Do I prefer serving with a team or by myself? Am I more introverted or extroverted?

If meditation peaks your interest, you may want to try out one of the hundreds of meditation ideas from Madonna Gauding, author of *The Meditation Bible*. She generated her meditations from a variety of ancient and modern traditions that are designed for many intentions. Taoism, along with Confucianism and Buddhism, is one of the three great religions of China. Lao-Tzu created a philosophy and way of life that is peaceful and in harmony with nature. Taoism has included acupuncture, holistic medicine, and martial arts. Here is one of Gauding's summarized meditation practices called "The Taoist Way":

> When: Practice this mediation when you want to feel more in harmony with nature and others.
>
> Preparation: Find a river or stream.
>
> 1. Sit or stand next to a river or stream at a spot where you can be quiet and undisturbed. Breathe deeply for a few minutes to quiet your mind.
> 2. Notice how the water flows over and around rocks or tree roots. Contemplate how life is more harmonious when you do not resist it or go against it.
> 3. Contemplate how you feel when trying to force an issue or make something happen according to your wishes.
> 4. Observe the stream and how water flows by choosing the path of least resistance. How can you use this wisdom of nature to make your life and the lives of those around you more peaceful and harmonious?

Face Your Mistakes

Enter the interview book that my business partners, Debby Bitticks and Lynn Benson, created called *Cherished Memories: The Story of My Life*. We were working on the final pieces of this amazing book and preparing it for quality control before our first appearance on QVC. I knew this book was a valuable tool for obtaining a loved one's life story, and I knew all the features and benefits about which I would speak while selling it on air—it is an excellent book. A few months before my training session with QVC hosts, and before getting our appointed spot on the QVC channel, it became clear that I needed to use this book with someone important to ensure my own and the book's credibility.

So I set out to meet with my mother over the course of several Sunday mornings to ask her the tenderly developed interview questions in the book. The book is divided into sections by age development (childhood days, teen years, early adulthood, and so on) with questions about your health history and an ethical will (the values you wish to pass on to your children); plus it has pockets to store memorabilia. Being the type-A person that I am, I started at the very beginning. From the moment I asked my mother the very first question, I realized I had never taken the time to learn her life story. Up until then I simply "endured" her regular stories whenever she decided to mention them. I was neither interested in nor appreciative about her past. I am embarrassed to admit this.

Just the act of taking an interest in my mother began to shift how I related to her. She did nothing different in the weeks ahead; she was just her usual self. But I was changing—and I hadn't even apologized yet. During our third breakfast meeting, I asked my mother a rather simple question from the book about her twelve-year-old life. Then it happened: My mom told me a story I hadn't heard before, and thank goodness I was truly interested in listening.

She said, "Well, Dorothy, I really wasn't having any fun at that age. I'm not sure we even went to school consistently. Living in Germany, my father had not come back from the war (he was presumed dead), and my mother was left with us—her five children— in tow. Our house was bombed in Berlin and we all had to walk for miles to live in a makeshift tent city in Czechoslovakia. We lost the few valuables we had, we took overcrowded trains, we were made to cross rushing rivers via a temporary swinging rope bridge, and each of us were separated and sent to temporary homes in other countries until the war was over." I gulped and continued to listen. My mother went on to tell the nightmarish details of bombs that looked like fireworks in the night sky and how her back would freeze at the sound of another air raid siren, and she finished her story by sharing what it was like to return once the war was over.

"Each of us children were assigned a chore in what was left of our bombed-out home. My job was to cook the family meals, since my mother worked during the day," said my mom about her mother. "I didn't know how I would make a meal. I was twelve years old. We had very little food and no stove. Later that day, I went outside and found an iron gutter grate dislodged in the street. I took the grate home, washed it, and turned it upside down and made a grill, and made the family meal." Mother told me this story so matter-of-factly. I sat there stunned with my eyelids blinking repeatedly. Let's see, at age twelve I was concerned about which color fuzzy pom-pom I would tie to the top of my roller skate next Friday night. I was seeing my mother in a whole new way; I was humbled, impressed, embarrassed, and proud. Something was about to change.

The next week, my mom and I prepared to have breakfast and continue with her life interview. I caught her in the garage doing laundry, and when I looked at her, I didn't see my mom. Instead, I saw this young child laboring over laundry. Every time I looked at my mother, I kept envisioning this sweet, innocent twelve-year-old, often frightened and always working, back in Berlin—conducting a life of struggle that even seasoned adults shouldn't have to contend with. My feelings were all too much. Where a week ago, I had little compassion for my mother, I suddenly had it now. Where previously I had found annoying what seemed to me to be my mother's endless questioning, it now appeared to be her way of caring and trying to relate to me. What used to agitate me about her suspicious nature was now obvious to me: my mother was just protecting herself from the fears of her past. I suddenly had the chance to see my mother for the innovative and creative spirit that she is. I stopped the interview to apologize to her.

She may not remember that day in the garage, but I do. It was a day when I grew up and said the things to a parent that adult children can hopefully find a way to say. Here are just a few of the apologies I made to my mom:

1. I'm sorry I didn't include you in the many family gatherings we arranged. I didn't think you would want to come, and sometimes it seemed too hard emotionally. I was wrong, and I'm sorry.

2. I used to drive fast when I was in my late teens. You were in the passenger seat and I remember you asking me to slow down. You were looking out for our safety. I took it to mean you were telling me what to do. I was stubborn. I didn't slow down. I'm sorry.

3. When I dated and later married a man twice my age, you questioned me and you warned me. I told you it was none of your business. He wasn't the right man for me. I'm sorry I didn't listen.

4. When I was 200-plus pounds, you delicately shared your concern, cooked healthy meals when we were together, and shared your own approach for staying healthy. I thought you were just hounding me. You weren't. You cared. I didn't hear you. I'm sorry.

Through my tears of shame, more apologies surfaced. I don't know where all of these words came from; they flowed through me like a rushing river about to crest after a rainstorm. My experience with the *Cherished Memories* book not only cleared the path for healing with my mother and positioned me to shave off the emotional and physical weight gain I was enduring, but it also set me and my business partner up for a complete sellout of our book on QVC. I'm especially glad I tested it out. So, who's next? I've got more work to do!

How Apologizing Ties Back to
Food and Weight Loss

As I do this weight-loss experiment, which includes looking at my shortcomings and past mistakes (intentional or unintentional) toward others, I can see a direct correlation: the more people I apologize to, the more weight falls off my body, and the more peace I have in my heart and my head (which keeps me from eating!). Did I mention I took off more than seventy-five pounds? That's a lot of apologizing.

Author Beverly Engle is a marriage, family, and child psychotherapist and the author of eighteen self-help books. She is an expert in the fields of sexual abuse, women's issues, relationships, and sexuality. In her amazing book *The Power of Apology: Healing Steps to Transform All Your Relationships*, she lists the many benefits to an apology, which were also published in the article "The Power of Apology" on the Psychology Today website at www.psychologytoday.com (July 1, 2002).

From my perspective of how apologies relate to weight loss, Engle shares how to give and receive an apology—and the impact it has on our health:

> Apology changed my life. I believe it can change yours as well. Almost like magic, apology has the power to repair harm, mend relationships, soothe wounds, and heal broken hearts. Apology is not just a social nicety. It is an important ritual, a way of showing respect and empathy for the wronged person. It is also a way of acknowledging an act that, if otherwise left unnoticed, might compromise the relationship. Apology has the ability to disarm others of their anger and to prevent further misunderstandings. While an apology cannot undo harmful past actions, if done sincerely and effectively, it can undo the negative effects of those actions. Apology is crucial to our mental and even physical health. Research shows that receiving an apology has a

noticeable, positive physical effect on the body. An apology actually affects the bodily functions of the person receiving it—blood pressure decreases, heart rate slows, and breathing becomes steadier.

Organizing Tips on Making Apologies

Making a list of my mistakes and identifying who may have been impacted by my mistakes was the beginning of my unloading a bunch of weight—physically and figuratively—from my body. A list of names of people to whom I owed an apology really did make a difference in my life, body, heart, and self-esteem. If you were to pick just one significant person with whom you could have this kind of conversation, I promise that your world would change. No blame, no fights, just a simple, "Do you remember when? I think I made a mistake. I'm sorry. I will avoid making this mistake again in the future." Aaron Lazare, MD, is chancellor, dean, and professor of psychiatry at the University of Massachusetts Medical School. He is a leading authority on the medical interview, the psychology of shame and humiliation, and apology. His most recent book is titled *On Apology*. He writes,

> There are up to four parts to an effective apology, though not every apology requires all four parts.
> 1. A valid acknowledgment of the offense that makes clear who the offender is and who is the offended. The offender must clearly and completely acknowledge the offense.
> 2. An effective explanation, which shows an offense was neither intentional nor personal, and is unlikely to recur.
> 3. Expressions of remorse, shame, and humility, which show that the offender recognizes the suffering of the offended.
> 4. A reparation of some kind, in the form of a real or symbolic compensation for the offender's transgression.

Sandy Brewer, PhD, author of the book *Pursuit of Light: An Extraordinary Journey* and host of the popular call-in talk radio show *The Sandy Brewer Show*, is a human behavior and relationship expert with more than thirty-five years' experience in the field of personal and professional growth and development. On her website, www.pursuitoflight.com, which is filled with informative articles, Dr. Brewer writes about forgiveness:

> We all have stories, but they are just backstories. Backstories can control and ruin our lives if we don't learn how to let them go. We are not our experiences; we are not the places through which we have traveled; and we are definitely not the result of someone else's ignorance and depravity. Unless we say so.
>
> Whatever one's life journey has been, we have the power within us to choose the challenges as stumbling blocks or stepping-stones. So, here's where forgiveness comes in, because no one can thrive as a victim. If we want freedom, joy, and laughter, if we want to create loving, caring relationships, if we want to know the parts of life we haven't yet known, then forgiveness—letting go of our attachment to our stories—is required. No healing, empowerment, or forward progress can happen without it. It takes courage to choose something greater than a wound, but we all have the power to do so. It is innate within us.
>
> So I chose that I was not a victim of the world around me or within me. I chose that I didn't have to stay afraid of what I had experienced. And I chose that I didn't have to sanitize it—to cover it with a pretty yellow ribbon or an endless shroud of grief. That would simply have kept me in fear of it and the frequency or energy that it represented. We do not change our lives or our world by sanitizing the harsh things we see or have seen. We create change by gaining strength, courage, wisdom, and conviction through looking the situation/energy of it in the eye and insisting that it does not name us. That falls under our jurisdiction! Forgiveness is about letting go

in peace, whether we are forgiving ourselves or others. It does not mean you are a dirty, rotten excuse for a human being and I forgive you anyway—even if the other person has behaved like a dirty rotten excuse for a human being. . . . Forgiveness is about compassion and release. It's about knowing that it takes two for war and one for peace. And in the end, forgiveness is understanding that from a spiritual point of view, there is nothing to forgive.

The art of forgiveness is, at its core, a release. It's the release of identifying oneself based on old stories; it's the cracking open of a once-wounded heart, the expansion of love. Each of us has the ability to discover the light and the promise of a new day if we will just let go of the idea that our identities have to be seeded in yesterday and willingly practice the healing art of forgiveness. That is how we create a today different than yesterday, for with each new dawn comes the light of a healed heart. Inner peace or inner war . . . which will you choose today?

6

UNSTUFFED:
Get Inspired
to Implement Your
Own Action Plan

Ladies and gentlemen, this is one area—and I've saved it for last—where there is no "before and after." There is no "how it was then, and how it is now" story. My entire life has been one goal after another, one dream followed by the next. I love where I've finally landed in my life. According to Lady Gaga, "Baby, I was born this way." Setting up an action plan is where my heart beats and my passion persists, not just for me but especially for others. The only thing that's different for me now is I'm doing it minus seventy-five pounds of physical weight and mind clutter. I can't imagine what my life would have been like if I didn't have to manage all of the pain, embarrassment, never-ending food thoughts and dieting associated with being overweight. But then again, I would not have the wealth of experiences I do now to relate to those who are still suffering.

As a child I used to play dress up and explore. Is it possible that reality TV was born inside my little head? My mother's bedroom was my *Project Runway* where I tried on my mother's high-heeled shoes, used towels as turbans, necklaces as tiaras, and sheets and blankets as royal robes. Near the clear-running stream in the back of our house was my *American Idol* stage where I sang to my audience: the cows in the field. At home, I built lavish tent rooms in the living room, tree houses outside, and over at my friend's house, too (just like on HGTV's *Trading Spaces*). When I hiked with other kids in the rolling hills out back, my hikes turned into a show similar to *Survivor*—I would make up games, tasks, and adventures for us to accomplish along the way. *Dancing with the Stars* happened many nights in our farmhouse-style dining room, where I created exotic costumes I'd seen and copied from the *Child Craft* books my parents bought for our studying. My family applauded, critiqued, and handed out awards. Heaven knows that none of these reality shows were on the air in the late 1960s; they were just little imaginary games and dreams inside my head. Even then I had dreams that ran along the lines of the impossible. And today? Well, now that's my job—helping others achieve their dreams through organization and personal coaching. I wonder, can we in fact look back to our childhood days to find what made us so gleeful then and see if those early activities could potentially reignite our goals and dreams again as adults?

When I turned twenty-one, I decided formally that I would do whatever I could to develop and achieve my dreams. Every year in January since then, I have a standing appointment with myself (friends and family have been included from time to time) to have an elegant afternoon tea at a very exclusive hotel and write my goals and action plan for the coming year. Having done this for nearly thirty years now, I can assure you that it works. The very act of writing down your goals gives you an increased chance of achieving them. Placing them in your calendar—like it's on your list of appointments to keep—nearly ensures it. My early goals were grand: to write books, travel the world, see the pyramids of Egypt, appear on a national talk show, speak a new language, take singing lessons, drive a Jaguar, pet a panda, meet the president of the United States, work on a hit TV show, attend Wimbledon, watch the Super Bowl in person, organize certain celebrity clients, try rock climbing, stay overnight in a castle, swim in secret waterfalls in Fiji. Those goals may have been grand, but the action plans were real, and I can look back on thirty years' worth of lists now and see how those wishes, fantasies, and grand ideas became realities. I've been able to enjoy all of them for real.

My goals and dreams still fuel me and inspire me. Yes, I have over-the-top goals for sure, but not as many. In fact, most goals and dreams are far less grand. I want to spend more time with my mom and my dear friends, brother, and sisters. I aspire to meditate at unique vista points in nature; I search for bright and sparkly gel pens to color in finely detailed coloring books designed for adult artists. When I hear about a comet coming through, I want to see it, and I now keep track of when the sun sets and watch the sun go down when I can.

It's hard to say which will inspire you more: facing your stuff so you can live your dreams or whether creating your dreams will motivate you to face your stuff. I think every individual responds differently; the key is to understand which way works for you. No matter what, generating new dreams, making an action plan, writing them down, and then discussing them with others will create a positive shift in your life.

Creating Your Action Plan

Name: _____

Today's Date: _____

Weight: _____

Stuffing It: Your Own Story

Where can you come clean about your past? This doesn't have to be long and involved, but writing your thoughts about why your life isn't working the way you want it to is incredibly valuable. Remember, small steps. Just a few sentences. Avoid perfection. Just write a little something:

_____

_____

_____

_____

_____

_____

Facing It:
Weight Loss or Food Addiction

Here's where you get clear about whether you think you have non-addictive problems losing weight or whether you might have a food obsession.

Motivate Yourself First

Decide now on action steps about your health and body, and list immediate solutions for them, starting with creating your goals and dreams. Here's the important part, the key to making this personalized action plan different from any others you've tried before, is to schedule the goals and dreams. Get out your calendar. Put these goals and dreams in your calendar, spaced out evenly throughout the year.

List two things you can do to improve your health or fitness in the coming year:

_____ log in to calendar

_____ log in to calendar

List two recreational activities you might want to try in the coming year:

_____ log in to calendar

_____ log in to calendar

Educationally, do you have an interest in learning anything new? If so, list it here:

_____ log in to calendar

_____ log in to calendar

Regarding family and friends, is there anyone who needs a little more attention from you? Do you feel the need to contact a long-lost friend? Do you need to practice saying no a little more to someone? Do you want to increase time with someone you really enjoy being around or maybe even decrease contact with someone who is a bit toxic?

_____ log in to calendar

_____ log in to calendar

Your wardrobe: Do you need anything, or do you want to get rid of anything?

_____ log in to calendar

_____ log in to calendar

If you are currently working, what would you like to change about your physical environment or perhaps your own attitude?

_____ log in to calendar

_____ log in to calendar

Does your home/flat/condo need repair? Do you need to purchase something? Need to get rid of anything? List a couple of goals to support your living environment.

_____ log in to calendar
_____ log in to calendar

Spirituality: Do you want more of it? Less of it? Want to learn about it? What could make you feel more spiritual?

_____ log in to calendar
_____ log in to calendar

Finances: Are you overspending in any area? Do you need to start a new savings account? Have you thought about talking to a financial planner?

_____ log in to calendar
_____ log in to calendar

Understand Your Mission

If you've read through most of this book, you will likely be able to decide for yourself whether you have to lose some weight because things have recently been a little out of control for you, or whether you feel you have an addiction to food. It is written in the inspirational book *Food for the Soul* "that a dose of sugar registers in the non-addict's brain as a little feather tickle, a pleasant sensation—but not a source of extreme stimulation igniting cravings, obsession, and compulsion." Decide now and take action.

- I need to lose weight.
- I think I may have a food obsession.

Start Practicing One New
Behavior Now—Pick Just One

If you feel you need a few tips to jump-start your weight loss, go back to the section about Organizing Tips for Healthy Eating and Exercise and review. If you feel you may have a food addiction, go back to that section and consider getting into a 12-step group at your first opportunity. In the meantime, take just *one small step*. Pick an idea from the suggestions below and take action.

- Clear your kitchen of any tempting foods.
- Keep your portion sizes steady, regular, and unchanging. Teach your stomach to expect the same amount of food at each meal. Drastic portion swings create cravings and set your food barometer to want more.
- Eliminate the "I can figure it out myself" syndrome. Commit to engaging in meaningful conversations with others. Don't do it alone. Find a group of people who have similar goals as you and participate. Pick up the phone, Google a group, step out of your comfort zone.
- Declare yourself! Declaring and organizing tomorrow's food today can be a total game changer. Deciding what you plan to eat tomorrow gives your brain a chance to figure out how to access healthy foods. Planning eradicates old patterns of vending-machine lunches and drive-through dinners. Plan it today. Live it tomorrow. Write down your food and follow through.
- Reach into the bowl! Cut a piece of paper into ten pieces. Write a different activity that you enjoy doing on each piece of paper. Crumple up the paper and toss it into the bowl, hat, or basket. When bored, rather than reach for a bowl of chips, reach for the surprise activity in the bowl instead. Break the cycle of boredom and create a new cycle of creativity and accomplishment.

- Just today, decide to get in touch with a Higher Power, Universal Power, or God. Have you ever thought of turning to prayer or meditation to help relieve you of food obsessions and cravings? Before you go down the path of overeating, try a quick spiritual break instead.

Facing It:
Tackling the Clutter Problem

Too much stuff can be one of the largest signals that we are avoiding something. Read about clutter (and hoarding) and its relationship to food, and find out if you can unearth your stuff in order to get your right-size body back.

Step 1

If Your Clutter Could Talk: It's your turn to write down what you think your clutter is saying. There really is a conversation behind—or under—all of it. Take a chance; reveal the secret of your clutter here. What is it saying? Be honest! Be bold!

_____

_____

_____

_____

_____

Now here's the cool part: You can decide right now what you would rather have your stuff say about you. When you walk through the door of your home or office, what do you want that space to say about you? Just jot down a few words that represent what/who you really see under all that clutter. These words will be the guiding motivation to a clutter-free space.

_____

_____

_____

_____

_____

_____

Step 2

Prioritize your problem areas. Here is a list of the most common areas of disorganization. Find the top ten areas that need the most attention from you and number them in order of importance. Some areas may not even be a problem for you. The point is that you want to look at these areas and ask yourself which one(s) bother you the most, cause you the most anxiety, or keep you from achieving a successful and healthy life. Spend less than three minutes on this. Your subconscious really knows what needs to be handled first—follow that inner voice.

_____ Addresses or contact info	_____ Jewelry
_____ Attic	_____ Junk drawer
_____ Basement	_____ Keys
_____ Bathroom	_____ Kids' artwork
_____ Books	_____ Kids' toys
_____ Closets	_____ Kitchen
_____ Clothes	_____ Living room
_____ Craft room	_____ Magazines
_____ Den	_____ Memorabilia
_____ Desk	_____ Office
_____ Dining room	_____ Paper
_____ Garage	_____ Patio
_____ Important documents	_____ Photographs

Once you have selected your top priority,

1. Pull up your calendar.
2. Make an appointment to work on the space or project.
3. Arrange for someone to help you.
4. Reread the steps about your chosen priority area in the Tackle Clutter section of this book to help you get started and stay on track.
5. Keep the project small and use a timer. Build on successful organizing sessions rather than give up because you tried to take on too much.

Facing It:
Banish Your Emotional Clutter

Sometimes it's not just the food or lack of exercise, but rather the emotional stuff that drives us to overeat. Which one will you take on? Next to each of the emotional clutter areas below, write down a response from your own life if you have one.

Emotional Clutter	Your Specific Issue	What You Really Want Instead
Face Your Failures	Example: I left my book club.	Example: I want to rejoin and be part of the group.
Face Your Fears and Anxieties	Example: I get anxiety when I open bills.	Example: I want to open my bills with ease.
Face Your Lack of Self-Esteem	Example: I'm jealous of Leanne.	Example: I want to smile more so I'm more approachable; Leanne does that.
Face Your Feelings	Example: I feel guilty most of the time.	Example: I need to learn to say no and feel okay about it.
Face Your Toxic Relationships	Example: Jim criticizes me way too often.	Example: I want to see a therapist so that I can nurture and take care of myself.

Honestly addressing these areas of life is one way to break down the barriers for retaining weight. It's usually the "stuff" on the inside of our heads that causes us to pack on the pounds on the outside of our bodies. Now that you have come to terms with some of your emotional clutter, it's time to select the area that you wish to address first.

Emotional clutter area I plan to address first:

_____

First step I will take to help myself in this area:

_____

Facing It: Curb the Chaos of Life

There are clues in life that can help you detect the reasons why you may consume too much food or the wrong kinds of food. You just know it when you look at the list below; one of these external life factors is staring at you more than the rest. Which is it? You may have been avoiding facing it for a long time, but you can take charge today. Put a check mark next to the subject that needs your attention first.

- Face your lack of sleep.
- Face your overwhelmed state (emotional/physical).
- Face your lack of time.
- Face your lack of finances.
- Face your isolation.

Now that you have selected your priority in terms of curbing your chaos, think about saying no. Saying no usually means we have to call in our very adult self to say no to our overdoing it. Let me explain:

Sleep	Say no to late-night television or projects.
Overwhelmed state	Say no to outside requests. Think before you respond.
Time	Say no to "I need to just do one more thing." That one more thing is probably the difference between your being late or showing up on time. It's all about discipline.
Finances	Say no to unplanned purchases. It's the compulsive buys that really throw our finances into chaos.
Isolation	Say no to another weekend afternoon home alone. Community can shift our sense of value and feeling of belonging.

The area of life I want to shift is _____
and I will do this by taking the following action _____
_____ on _____
(list the date you intend to take the action).

Ladies and gentlemen, my story is not terribly significant. There are folks in the world (perhaps you) who have suffered far greater circumstances than me and performed far more heroic acts than I have. There are surgeons who reattach limbs, pilots who safely land planes destined for disaster, firefighters, EMTs, and Coast Guard responders who save lives in seconds—and sometimes lose their own doing it. There are caregivers who soften the pain and mothers who champion the cause against bullying. There is nothing special about me or my story, except that I have figured some things out—some things that may matter in another human being's life, maybe even yours.

I thank you for taking the time to read parts or all of this book. My journey continues, and by no means am I guaranteed glory and success, but I can finally say, "I know better, I will act better, and I want to be better." I had a lot to learn, and perhaps I learned it for you or someone you know. Whether it's an obsession with food or issues with self-esteem, whether you're struggling with your finances or too much clutter, whether you're in need of a community or need to commune with God, I want to let you know it takes only a small step to get started. Just *one little, itty-bitty step*. Please say you'll try. Please say you will finally *face your stuff.* Good luck, and avoid perfection at all costs!

MORE FROM DOROTHY THE ORGANIZER:

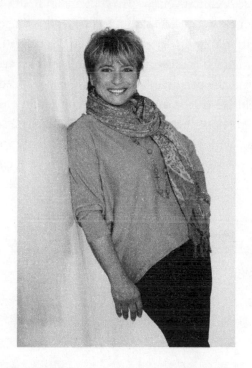

Personal or Business Coaching

Dorothy Breininger works with you to understand your areas of challenge and stress, your goals and needs, and helps you develop a step-by-step organizational action plan to achieve your dreams.

Toll Free: 1-888-229-5346

E-mail: info@DorothyTheOrganizer.com

Face Your Stuff System

Whether you're a pack rat or a calorie counter, a neat freak or a binge eater, to be successful on the scale, you must first master the clutter within you and around you. The Face Your Stuff System gives you the tools to declutter your way to your dream size by transforming and adopting new ways of thinking, feeling, and acting differently by facing the stuff in your life. Let Dorothy the Organizer be your coach and mentor to guide you every step of the way. This system teaches you how to take the necessary steps with a personalized action plan, access to exclusive videos, and a support community to help ensure that your weight-loss dreams become a reality. Every Face Your Stuff System comes with a thirty-day money-back guarantee. For more information, please visit www.FaceYourStuffSystem.com.

MEET THE AUTHOR

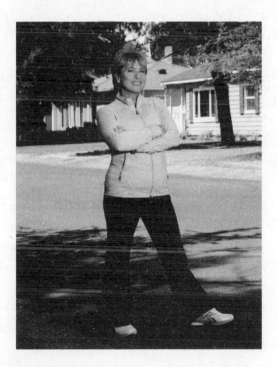

Dorothy Breininger is America's most innovative professional organizer, and she is on a mission to create more space on the planet. Dorothy is past president of NAPO Los Angeles, served on the board of directors for NAPO, and is a member and lecturer for the Institute for Challenging Disorganization (ICD). Dorothy is one of A&E® TV's expert organizers on the Emmy-nominated weekly TV series *Hoarders*.® She has also appeared on the *Today* show, the *Dr. Phil* show, *The View*, QVC, and PBS, in addition to being featured in the *Wall Street Journal*, *Forbes*, and *Oprah*.

Dorothy founded the Delphi Center for Organization, which has thousands of clients ranging from corporations, celebrities, individuals, small businesses, and busy moms, and, of course, operates a hoarding division at the center to manage the exploding hoarding epidemic existing in Western cultures. Dorothy works very closely with local, state, and federal government agencies in terms of training and on-site hoarding remediation.

Dorothy coauthored *BioBinder Cherished Memories: The Story of My Life* (Delphi Health Products, 2011), *Time Efficiency Makeover* (2005), *The Senior Organizer* (2006), and *Life Lessons for Busy Moms: 7 Essential Ingredients to Organize and Balance Your World* (2007) with Jack Canfield and Mark Victor Hansen (all published by Health Communications, Inc.).

Dorothy produced and hosted a PBS television pledge special and the award-winning documentary *Saving Our Parents*, starring Ed Asner, Art Linkletter, and LAPD chief William Bratton. Dorothy is a high-energy, sought-after national speaker who inspires her audiences to produce results and take immediate action. She is the 2005 U.S. Small Business Association award winner and a three-time recipient of NAPO-L.A.'s "Most Innovative Organizer" award. Visit her website at www.DorothyTheOrganizer.com.

MEET THE CONTRIBUTORS

Dee Dee Wilson Barton (aka *The Dee View*) is a mother who is in a state of perpetual shock because she just didn't expect it to be this hard! A chick with a potty mouth, she loves martinis, parties, and kids who are quiet. A full-figured girl, she redefines Fat Chic while wearing very high heels or the world's most expensive orthopedic shoes. Dee Dee and her husband own a full-service accounting firm in Palm Springs, California. They are positive that they are Dorothy Breininger's favorite clients. Dee Dee has an opinion about everything and is dying to share it with you! Check out her book at http://tinyurl.com/TheDeeView.

MaryAnne Bennic is Australia's organizing guru and most prolific systems creator and author. Her systems offer people more time, money, and energy, but more important, give people a sense of control over their homes, their offices, and their lives. MaryAnne holds a bachelor's degree in education and a master's degree in business, and she created two trademarked systems: the Paper Flow system for managing paperwork and the in8steps system for managing and organizing space. Her two books, *Paper Flow: Your Ultimate Guide to Making Paperwork Easy* (2011, coauthored with Brigitte Hinneberg) and *From Stuffed to Sorted: Your Essential Guide to Organizing Room by Room* (2011), are bestsellers and provide lifesaving advice to people all over the world.

She has appeared on Lifestyle Television, in radio interviews, and in countless magazines and newspapers. As a sought-after presenter, trainer, and speaker, she inspires and motivates people to make positive changes to their lives. She is a Victorian Australasian Association of Professional Organisers (AAPO) forum leader and an active AAPO expert member who provides training to organizers from all over the world. Visit her website at www.in8.com.au.

Lynn Benson, "mommy expert" and president of Delphi Health Products, coauthored *BioBinder Cherished Memories: The Story of My Life* (Delphi Health Products, 2011) and *The Senior Organizer* (HCI, 2006). Prior to her position at Delphi, Lynn's career began in the child-care field. Starting off as a preschool teacher, she was then promoted to center director. Lynn eventually became a regional director, overseeing the operations of a national multiunit, intergenerational company that cared for children *and* elders. During this time, she spent countless hours creating and organizing systems to ensure the quality of the intergenerational curriculum and daily procedures. Lynn also has a master's degree in social work and a diverse and significant background working with children, families, and seniors. She is the mother of two young children. Visit her website at www.DelphiHealthProducts.com.

Debby Bitticks, a nationally recognized intergenerational expert and CEO of Delphi Health Products, coauthored *BioBinder Cherished Memories: The Story of My Life* (Delphi Health Products, 2011), and *Time Efficiency Makeover* (2005), *The Senior Organizer* (2006), and *Life Lessons for Busy Moms: 7 Essential Ingredients to Organize and Balance Your World* with Jack Canfield and Mark Victor Hansen (all published by Health Communications, Inc.). A recognized expert, Debby has presented and spoken at the National Council on Aging (NCOA) in Washington, DC, on intergenerational care, and she has appeared on CBS, NBC, ABC, Fox, CNN

Financial News, and other cable shows, as well as giving numerous national radio interviews. Debby also appeared on QVC with *Bio-Binder Cherished Memories: The Story of My Life*. Debby wrote and hosted a PBS television show and coproduced the award-winning documentary *Saving Our Parents*. Visit her website at www.DelphiHealthProducts.com.

Pat Brady has a diverse background in corporate communications, as well as serving as a lead copy editor for many *Chicken Soup for the Soul* authors. After Pat received a master's degree in education from Pepperdine University, she taught in many underserved communities and now operates a private tutoring company. She enthusiastically believes that all students can learn and uses differentiated teaching skills to ensure client success. Email her at TutoringWithPat@yahoo.com.

Sandy Brewer, PhD, host of the popular call-in talk radio show *The Sandy Brewer Show*, is a human behavior and relationship expert with over thirty-five years of experience in the field of personal and professional growth and development. Sandy, a renowned speaker, author, therapist, coach, and humanitarian, has captivated audiences from Pepperdine University (CA) to Alice Tully Hall at Lincoln Center (NYC) as well as internationally. She has been featured on numerous television shows, including NBC's *Nightly News*. A documentary on a special project Sandy founded to work with abused and traumatized children, called *A Bridge for the Children*, was televised nationally. Visit Dr. Brewer's website at www.pursuitoflight.com.

Dr. Margaret Christensen is a board-certified ob/gyn who received her undergraduate degree from Rice University in Houston, Texas, graduating cum laude with degrees in biology and psychology. She subsequently received her medical degree from Baylor College of

Medicine in Houston, graduating with high honors. She received her board certification as a fellow of the American College of Obstetrics and Gynecology and was recertified in 2003. In 2001 she was called by Spirit to close her traditional practice and take a two-year sabbatical for research, transformative growth, and profound personal healing. By integrating and applying her findings on creating health into her own life, she now helps inspire her clients to do the same in her new practice, the Christensen Center for Whole Life Health. Visit her website at www.christensencenter.com.

Gillian Drake is an independent contractor who wears many hats: office manager, researcher, and writer, as well as client, event, and public relations liaison. A former legal secretary and Body and Mind therapist, she believes that embracing all life's experiences—good and bad—can foster growth and positive change. A graduate of the Southern Universities Joint Board in England, Gillian has worked with Dorothy the Organizer and her partners at Delphi Digital, Inc., for nine years. Grateful for the opportunity to contribute to this project, she hopes that many will find valuable insights within these pages. Contact GillianPR@ymail.com.

Karen Koedding is Australia's first certified professional organizer (CPO) and the founder of A Little Elf, a professional organizing firm established in New York City, now based in Sydney, Australia. Karen's background includes financial management roles in large corporate and small start-up businesses. Helping her clients get organized gives them freedom from stress and allows for new energy in their lives and businesses. Her firm specializes in creating organized, functional, aesthetically pleasing spaces for clients. Karen is a Golden Circle member of the National Association of Professional Organizers (NAPO), an expert member of the Australasian Association of Professional Organizers (AAPO), and is a subscriber of the Institute for Challenging Disorganization. Karen provides business consulting for small and medium-size businesses and offers mentoring to new professional organizers, as well as webinars for experienced professional organizers. Visit her website at www.alittleelf.com and www.facebook.com/ALittleElf; or reach her at Ph +61 419 446 109; e-mail: info@alittleelf.com.

Veteran teacher, real estate developer, and world traveler **Timolin Langin,** aka "Timmie the Teacher," is from a small town in Mississippi. There, a generation of relatives with a "mother wit" for financial success taught her how humble earnings could yield a fiscal life stable enough to support all of her dreams, travel, and interests. No matter what your socioeconomic status is at the moment, Timmie can help you become a more effective money manager. She proves that financial success is less about income and more about good spending habits and diligent saving, because these simple philosophies apply to all salaries, whether $10,000 or $10 million per year. Please visit Timmie's website at www.NewFitWorldTV.com or call 213-453-3921.

Valentina Sgro is a member of the Golden Circle of the National Association of Professional Organizers (NAPO), a chronic disorganization specialist, and the owner of SGRO Consulting, Solutions for Getting *Really* Organized. She is the current president of the Institute for Challenging Disorganization. Val is an award-winning author who brings the world of professional organizing alive for readers in her novels and short stories, which feature protagonist Patience Oaktree. Contact Val at www.reallyorganized.com.

Kipling Solid holds a degree in corporate fitness and currently owns Solid Bodies, a personal training and Pilates studio. Kipling has combined experience of twenty-plus years in the fitness industry. She pioneered the personal fitness in-home training industry in 1990. She specializes in rehabilitation and competitive training and is a fully certified Pilates teacher. She has a background in classical ballet, modern dance, and bodybuilding. This experience has equipped her with a keen knowledge of movement and body alignment. Kipling has a dedicated lifelong commitment to healthy and joyful living. She resides in Highland Park, Illinois, with her two sons. She can be reached at Solid Bodies, personal training and Pilates studio: (847) 830-8659. www.kiplingpilates.com.

Charlene Underhill Miller, PhD, is a licensed marriage, family, and child therapist in California, professor, clinical supervisor, and popular public speaker. Dr. Miller provides psychotherapy to individuals, couples, and families. She treats a wide range of issues, such as relational problems, self-sabotage, and parenting challenges, as well as compulsive problems such as eating disorders, hoarding, and addictions, which often have their origins in trauma. An adjunct faculty member at Pepperdine University's Graduate School of Education and Psychology, Dr. Miller has also taught at Fuller Theological Seminary's School of Psychology and Azusa Pacific University's Graduate School of Psychology. Dr. Miller holds master's and PhD degrees in Marriage and Family Therapy from Fuller's School of Psychology, as well as a bachelor's degree in psychology from UCLA. Dr. Miller is a happy wife and a proud mother and stepmother—living in a houseful of boys and two dogs! Dr. Miller sees clients in Malibu, Santa Monica, and Pasadena, California. Visit her website at www.underhillmiller.com, or reach her at (310) 576-0883.

RESOURCES

Making a Difference for Others

Aid Still Required

"Just because it left the headlines doesn't mean it left the planet." Aid Still Required (ASR) champions forgotten issues and people who have been left behind after natural disasters and human crises and after the media spotlight has faded. ASR's awareness campaigns have reached more than 250 million people worldwide through collaborations with the world's most respected musicians, actors, and athletes, including Paul McCartney, Sting, Maroon 5, Bonnie Raitt, Usher, Alicia Keys, Kevin Spacey, Hugh Jackman, Kobe Bryant, Chris Paul, Steve Nash, Grant Hill, and Landon Donovan. Aid Still Required is currently focusing on New Orleans, Haiti, Darfur, and the region affected by the 2004 tsunami, all areas where disasters occurred years ago and where survivors are still very much in need. Please join me in helping those who have been left behind. A portion of these book sales will go to support this charity. Visit the website at www.AidStillRequired.org.

The Institute for Challenging Disorganization (ICD)

If you need help with your own or a loved one's hoarding situation, I suggest visiting this website. The ICD mission is to provide education, research, and strategies to benefit people challenged by chronic disorganization. You will also find hundreds and hundreds of professionals on this site. Once you input your country and ZIP code, you will find a host of individuals with specialized training in the world of challenging disorganization. Visit the website at www. challengingdisorganization.org.

National Association of Professional Organizers (NAPO)

If you need help organizing, your best bet is to visit this website. There are thousands and thousands of professional organizers all over the United States and the world who can help you in every aspect of organizing. In addition, many of these professional organizers are certified. Just as you can hire a CPA, now you can also hire a CPO (certified professional organizer). Just put in your ZIP code and check off the areas you want to get organized. You'll get a list of names back pronto. Visit the website at www.NAPO.net.

Twelve-Step Groups

AA	Alcoholics Anonymous
ACA	Adult Children of Alcoholics
Al-Anon/ Alateen	For friends and family members of alcoholics
CA	Cocaine Anonymous
CLA	Clutterers Anonymous
CMA	Crystal Meth Anonymous
Co-Anon	For friends and family of addicts
CoDA	Co-Dependents Anonymous *(for people working to end patterns of dysfunctional relationships and develop functional and healthy relationships)*

COSA	Formerly Known as Codependents of Sex Addicts
COSLAA	Co-Sex and Love Addicts Anonymous
DA	Debtors Anonymous
EA	Emotions Anonymous *(recovery from mental and emotional illness)*
EHA	Emotional Health Anonymous *(recovery from mental and emotional illness)*
FA	Families Anonymous *(for relatives and friends of addicts)*
FA	Food Addicts in Recovery Anonymous
FAA	Food Addicts Anonymous
GA	Gamblers Anonymous
Gam-Anon/ Gam-A-Teen	For friends and family members of problem gamblers
HA	Heroin Anonymous
MA	Marijuana Anonymous
NA	Narcotics Anonymous
NAIL	Neurotics Anonymous *(for recovery from emotional and mental illness)*
Nar-ANON	For friends and family members of addicts
NiCA	Nicotine Anonymous
OA	Overeaters Anonymous
OLGA	Online Gamers Anonymous
PA	Pills Anonymous *(for recovery from prescription pill addiction)*

SA	Sexaholics Anonymous
SA	Smokers Anonymous
SAA	Sex Addicts Anonymous
SCA	Sexual Compulsives Anonymous
SIA	Survivors of Incest Anonymous
SLAA	Sex and Love Addicts Anonymous
WA	Workaholics Anonymous

Books

I have personally found these books very helpful, among many others.

Davis, William. *Wheat Belly: Lose the Wheat, Lose the Weight, and Find Your Path Back to Health.* Emmaus, PA: Rodale, 2011.

Fuhrman, Joel. *Eat to Live: The Amazing Nutrient-Rich Program for Fast and Sustained Weight Loss.* Rev. ed. New York: Little, Brown and Co., 2011.

Hasselbeck, Elisabeth. *The G-Free Diet: A Gluten-Free Survival Guide.* New York: Center Street, 2009.

Lamm, Steven, and Sidney Stevens. *No Guts, No Glory: Gut Solution, the Core of Your Total Wellness.* Laguna Beach, CA: Basic Health Publications, 2012.

NOTES

Introduction

1. http://www.usatoday.com/story/news/nation/2013/01/07/decrease-dieting-weight/1814305/.

Chapter 4

1. http://en.wikipedia.org/wiki/Pygmalion_effect#Rosenthal-Jacobson study.

Chapter 5

1. http://greater good.berkeley.edu/expanding gratitude.

2. http://healthhub.brighamandwomens.org/research-meditation-and-the-dalai-lama; http://www.hms.harvard.edu/hmni/On_The_Brain/Volume12/OTB_Vol12No3_Fall06.pdf.

3. http://newsroom.ucla.edu/portal/ucla/evidence-builds-that-meditation-230237.aspx.

4. http://www.huffingtonpost.com/robert-e-herron-phd/transcendental-meditation_b_1671832.html

5. http://www.vancouversun.com/health/Meditation+helps+kids+attention+leading+researcher+says/6159558/story.html.

6. http://www.livestrong.com/article/26922-depression-cause-overeating.

INDEX